DIABETES INSIPIDUS

Edited by **Kyuzi Kamoi**

Diabetes Insipidus
Edited by Kyuzi Kamoi

Published by InTech
Janeza Trdine 9, 51000 Rijeka, Croatia

Notice
Statements and opinions expressed in the chapters are these of the individual contributors and not necessarily those of the editors or publisher. No responsibility is accepted for the accuracy of information contained in the published chapters. The publisher assumes no responsibility for any damage or injury to persons or property arising out of the use of any materials, instructions, methods or ideas contained in the book.

Publishing Process Manager Masa Vidovic

Technical Editor Teodora Smiljanic

Cover Designer InTech Design Team

Additional hard copies can be obtained from orders@intechopen.com

Diabetes Insipidus, Edited by Kyuzi Kamoi
p. cm.
ISBN 978-953-307-367-5

Meet the editor

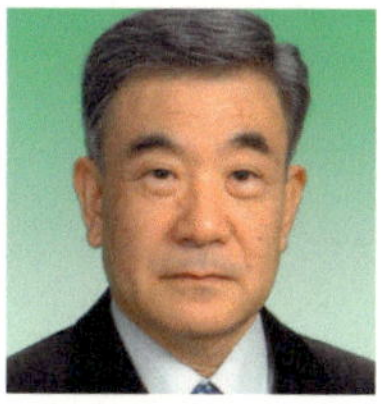

Professor Kyuzi Kamoi was born August 28, 1943 in Tokyo, Japan. He received his MD in 1970 and his MSD in 1982, both from the Medical School of Niigata University, Niigata, Japan. He has received the following certificates: Japan Medical Diplomat (1970), Japan Board of Diabetes Mellitus (1990), Japan Board of Endocrinology and Metabolism (1991), Certified Diabetes Mellitus Educator (1993), Certified Endocrine Educator (2004). From 1980 to 2010 he was Chief of Internal Medicine, and from 2002 until 2010 the Director of Center of Diabetes Mellitus and Endocrine Disease at Nagaoka Red Cross Hospital, Japan. Since 2010 to the present he has been Professor of Niigata Prefecture University. He is a member of The Japanese Society of Internal Medicine, The Japan Endocrine Society, The Japanese Society of Hypertension, The Japan Society of Hypertension, the Endocrine Society, The American Society of Hypertension, The American Diabetes Association, The International Diabetes Federation and the New York Academy of Science. He has published a total of 200 scientific papers.

Contents

Preface

This primary aim of this publication is to show recent scientific findings regarding clinical problems of diabetes insipidus (DI) to all readers.

In a clinical setting, DI is divided into 4 types which are consisted of neurogenic, nephrogenic, dipsogenic (primary polydipsia) and gestational types.

In 1794, DI was separated from diabetes mellitus by Dr. Frank JP who first defined DI in the world. After that, the investigation of pathophysiology in DI has proceeded with the development of science.

Secretions of blood vasopressin (AVP) are clarified by the developments of measuring method and more adequate test for AVP secretion. Moreover, the development of MRI imaging on the pituitary gland with the stalk and hypothalamus gives us more evidentiary information. Non-inflammatory diseases as pathophysiology of DI from idiopathic causes are elucidated and the pathophysiology of nephrogenic DI and gestational DI has been more clarified.

However, there are many unsolved problems in the field. For example, although adipsic DI in neurogenic types is a rare disorder, its management is difficult. The main factor may be caused by disturbance of the osmoreceptor. The osmoreceptor is a theoretical concept and is not yet concretely established by recent scientific developments. Further, it is crucial to measure plasma AVP in DI. However, as it is difficult to measure plasma AVP easily in the world, other methods except plasma AVP have been searched. Among the methods, there is hope in the measurement of plasma copeptin. Regarding clinical problems, differential diagnosis of autoimmune diseases with other causes is not easy. It needs to have a method for detecting the autoantibody for autoimmunity of DI simply and trustworthily. In the gene, although some types have demonstrated relation to gene abnormality, it is not clear to how the gene abnormality causes the DI.

The authors have contributed significant scientific findings and I hope that readers understand the recent pathophysiology of DI.

Prof. Kyuzi Kamoi
Niigata Prefecture University
Japan

1

Management of Langerhans Cell Histiocytosis (LCH)-Induced Central Diabetes Insipidus and Its Associated Endocrinological/Neurological Sequelae

Shinsaku Imashuku[1] and Akira Morimoto[2]
[1]*Division of Pediatrics, Takasago-seibu Hospital, Takasago,*
[2]*Department of Pediatrics, Jichi Medical University, Shimotsuke,*
Japan

1. Introduction

Central diabetes insipidus (CDI) is caused by a deficiency of arginine vasopressin (AVP), also known as antidiuretic hormone. Although CDI is rare in children and young adults, it should be kept in mind that it is associated with rare histiocytic disorders in the central nervous system (CNS), namely Langerhans cell histiocytosis (LCH), xanthogranulomatosis and Erdheim-Chester disease, all of which specifically affect the hypothalamus and pituitary stalk, thereby inducing CDI (**1,2**). In particular, CDI is the most frequently occurring CNS event in patients with multi-focal LCH, who often have multisystem lesions, including craniofacial bone lesions (**3**). LCH is a rare disorder that is characterized by the proliferation of cells that bear the activated Langerhans cell phenotype (**4**). Early studies reported that CDI occurs in 25–50% of LCH patients but this incidence appears to have dropped to 7–20% since the introduction of systemic chemotherapy (**5**). CDI can develop either before, simultaneously with, or subsequent to a diagnosis of LCH based on the presence of various extracranial lesions. It can also develop during chemotherapy for systemic LCH or after therapy. Patients with LCH-induced CDI show typical clinical symptoms, such as polyuria/polydispsia, in association with abnormal radiographic findings, such as a thickened pituitary stalk or a hypothalamic mass and the loss of a hot signal (T1 weighted) for the pituitary posterior lobe on brain magnetic resonance imaging (MRI) (**5-8**). Once CDI develops, it becomes irreversible in most patients, who will require life-long desmopressin replacement therapy with 1-desamino-8-D-arginine vasopressin(DDAVP). In addition, 30–58% of patients with CDI exhibit anterior pituitary hormone deficiencies (APHD) during follow-up (**1,7**). LCH-associated APHD appears to be linked to a thickening of the pituitary stalk (**6,7**). In addition, patients with LCH-induced CDI can eventually develop neurodegenerative (ND) disease (**9,10**).

Appropriate management of LCH-induced CDI involves (a) a prompt correct diagnosis; (b) early intervention with chemo/radiotherapy to reverse the CDI, if possible; (c) appropriately treating CDI to prevent the later development of APHD or ND disease; (d) good control of CDI, once it has become permanent, with DDAVP; and ideally (e) exploring future innovative measures that could prevent the occurrence of CDI in patients with LCH.

2. Diagnosis of LCH-related CDI

2.1 Risk factors associated with the development of CDI

CDI occurs most often among pediatric patients with multi-focal LCH, particularly those with multi-system disease with proptosis (**11**). Moreover, LCH lesions in the craniofacial bones are seen in >75% of CDI patients (**7**). We also found that LCH-induced CDI is associated significantly more frequently ($p<0.001$) with multi-system multi-focal bone lesions, particularly lesions in craniofacial bones (temporal bone, ear-petrous bone, orbita, and zygomatic bone), than with single system bone lesions (**12**).

2.2 Diagnosis of CDI

CDI is generally suspected on the basis of the characteristic symptoms of polyuria/polydipsia. To correctly diagnose CDI, the water deprivation with desmopression test has long been employed (**13,14**). At diagnosis, to confirm that CDI has developed, it is necessary to determine plasma osmolality (reference values, 276–292 mOsm/kg H_2O) together with plasma AVP levels (reference values, 0.3–4.2 pg/ml by RIA 2 antibody method). The plasma osmolarity, AVP, and water deprivation test data are important for the early diagnosis of partial CDI, which is critical for preventing the progression into permanent CDI. However, sequential plasma osmolarity, AVP, and water deprivation test data are not available from the pre-CDI period to partial CDI and to complete CDI phase for patients.

CDI may occur before, simultaneously with, or subsequent to a diagnosis of LCH that is made on the basis of biopsies of extra-cranial peripheral lesions such as those in the skin, bone, and soft tissues. The definite diagnosis of LCH is made on the basis of histopathology of granulomatous lesions that reveals the presence of CD1a-, Langerin (CD207)- and S100-positive cells (**15**). If the initial and only lesion in patients with CDI is a thickened stalk, it may be necessary to biopsy the stalk since it has been reported that pituitary stalk thickening precedes the typical peripheral lesions of LCH by several months (**16**). However, the decision to biopsy should be made carefully, but it must be done promptly. The diagnosis and treatment of such cases are often delayed because physicians tend to follow a "wait and see" policy.

2.3 Differential diagnosis

CDI has various etiologies. Some are idiopathic while others are mass lesions on the hypothalamic-pituitary axis caused by germinoma, histiocytic disorders (including LCH), trauma, or inflammatory or infectious diseases (**1,2,17,18).** According to a large study by Maghnie *et al.*(**1**), the etiologies in 52% of CDI cases were idiopathic, while LCH accounted for another 15%. It should be noted that LCH should be suspected first in children with CDI, and that about 70% show pituitary stalk thickening while the remaining 30% may demonstrate a hypothalamic mass. In contrast, in adults, CDI is more frequently caused by inflammatory processes such as sarcoidosis or tuberculosis and neoplastic infiltrations that do not originate from neuronal tissue (**2**). Another possible cause in adults is lymphocytic hypophysitis, which is also termed infundibulo-neurohypophysitis or lymphocytic infundibulo-neurohypophysitis (**19**). Whenever this is suspected, the diagnosis is often delayed because a "wait and see" policy is adopted; this is because the disease is thought to be essentially self-limited.

2.4 Radiographic findings

Abnormal radiographic findings that are associated with CDI are a thickened pituitary stalk or hypothalamic mass and the loss of a hot signal (on T1-weighted MRI) in the pituitary posterior lobe (**Figure 1, 2**). According to Grois *et al.* (**7**), by the time CDI is diagnosed in LCH patients, 71% already exhibit a thickened stalk, while MRIs performed more than 5 years after CDI onset show that the stalk is still thickened in 24% of patients. Also, in a small percentage of patients, the stalk was already thickened several months before CDI onset. In addition, in the study of Maghnie *et al.* (**1**), where CDI cases with various etiologies were reviewed, 37% exhibited thickening of the pituitary stalk on the first MRI scan and, in 94%, the posterior pituitary was not hyper-intense. Moreover, when the course of CDI was examined in 18 patients who had a normal or thickened pituitary stalk at presentation, changes in the thickness of the stalk were observed over time: these included normalization, a decrease in thickness, further thickening, and thickening of a previously normal stalk
Regarding the loss of the hot spot in the posterior pituitary lobe, we have often found it difficult to interpret the T1-weighted MRI findings because the hot signal in the posterior lobe is masked or overlapped by the hot signal of the dorsum sellae. This problem can be overcome if the slice on MRI is performed appropriately so that the posterior pituitary and the dorsum sellae are separated (**8,20**) (**Figure 1**). The high signal in the posterior lobe is due to the retention of AVP (**8**), while the high signal in the dorsum sellae reflects the dura membrane that covers the thin bony dorsum sellae. It has been suggested that the fat suppression technique and a horizontal direction of frequency encoding could help to differentiate the high signal of the neurohypophysis from that of the dorsum sella (**20**). In

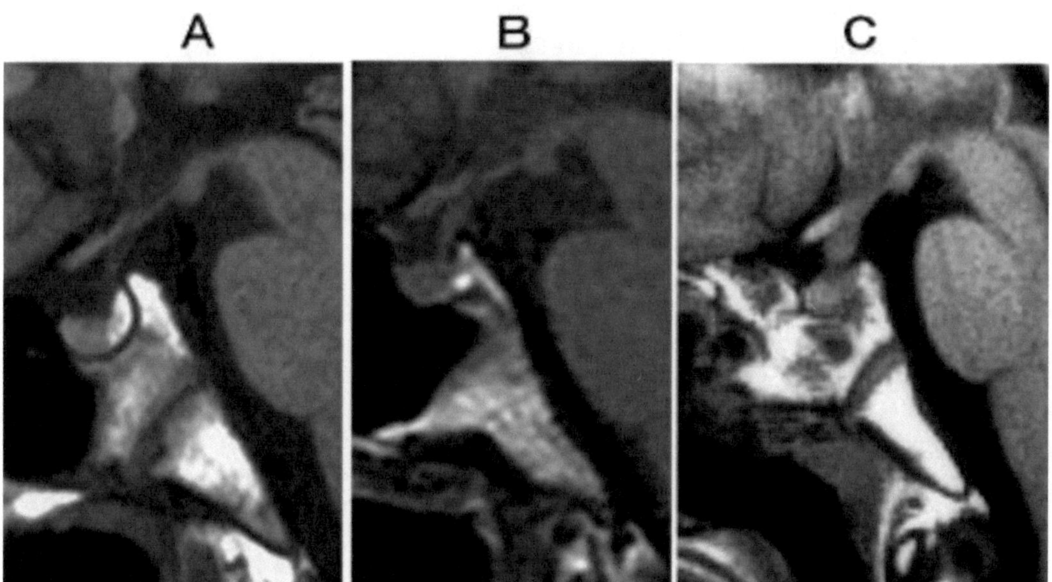

Fig. 1. MRI reveals normal and abnormal hypothalamic-pituitary regions. In two healthy controls, a hot signal in the pituitary lobe that is clearly separated from the dorsum sella can be observed (**A,B:** T1-weighted). A patient with LCH shows a thickened stalk and the loss of the hot spot in the posterior lobe (**C:** T1-weighted).

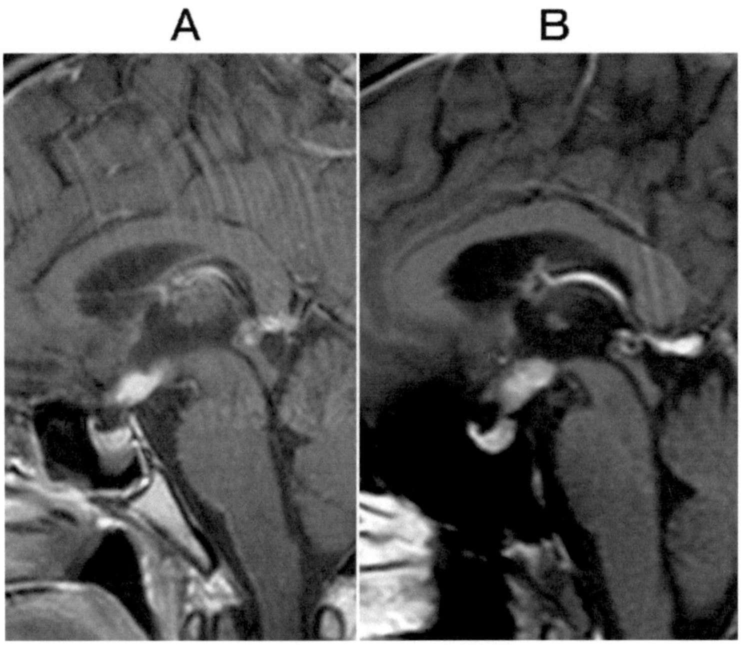

Fig. 2. Gadolinium-enhanced MRIs show a hypothalamic mass in two patients with LCH (**A, B**), each of which was histopathologically confirmed to be LCH by biopsy.

addition, it is recommended that to confirm the diagnosis of CDI in patients with polyuria/polydipsia, an early survey of the hypothalamic-pituitary axis by Gadolinium-enhanced MRI should be performed (**Figure 2**).

2.5 CDI-related CNS complications - Anterior Pituitary Hormone Deficiencies (APHD) and Neurodegenerative (ND) Disease

LCH-induced hypopituitarism has been described in children as well as in adults **(21-24)**. Clinically, the symptoms start with CDI and then progress to anterior pituitary dysfunction, particularly growth hormone insufficiency. The 10-year risk of developing growth hormone deficiency is 54% in pediatric patients (**25**). However, sex hormone deficiency or hypogonadism has also been reported in both adult-onset cases of LCH and adults with childhood-onset LCH. Kaltsas *et al.*(**23**) found that at a median of 4.5 yr after the diagnosis of CDI in 12 adult cases, eight exhibited growth hormone deficiency, seven had FSH-LH deficiency, five showed TSH/ACTH deficiency, and five had panhypopituitarism. Similarly, in ten pediatric LCH cases with CDI, Amato *et al.*(**24**) reported growth hormone deficiency in four, obesity in three, and hypogonadism in two. Moreover, Maghnie *et al.* (**1**) found that the prevalence of growth hormone deficiency after the onset of CDI was 61% at a median of 0.6 year after onset (range, 0.1 to 18.0). In advanced cases, panhypopituitarism develops.

LCH-associated ND disease develops in 1–4% of LCH patients **(9,10)** but the correlation between CDI and ND disease is not as clear as the correlation between CDI and APHD. Grois *et al.* (**7**) reported that 76% of CDI patients with follow-up MRIs performed at least 5 years after diagnosis exhibited neurodegenerative brain changes, showing a correlation between CDI and ND disease. On the other hand, we have noted in Japan that 50% of patients with LCH-induced ND disease had CDI but the other half did not (**10**). MRI is the most sensitive and commonly used technique for the diagnosis and monitoring of lesions in the cerebellum and basal ganglia (**Figure 3**). Symptomatic patients with this disorder show neurological dysfunction such as clumsiness, tremor, dysarthria, dysphagia, nystagmus, dysmetria and ataxia (**9,10**). The eventual outcome of ND disease is dismal.

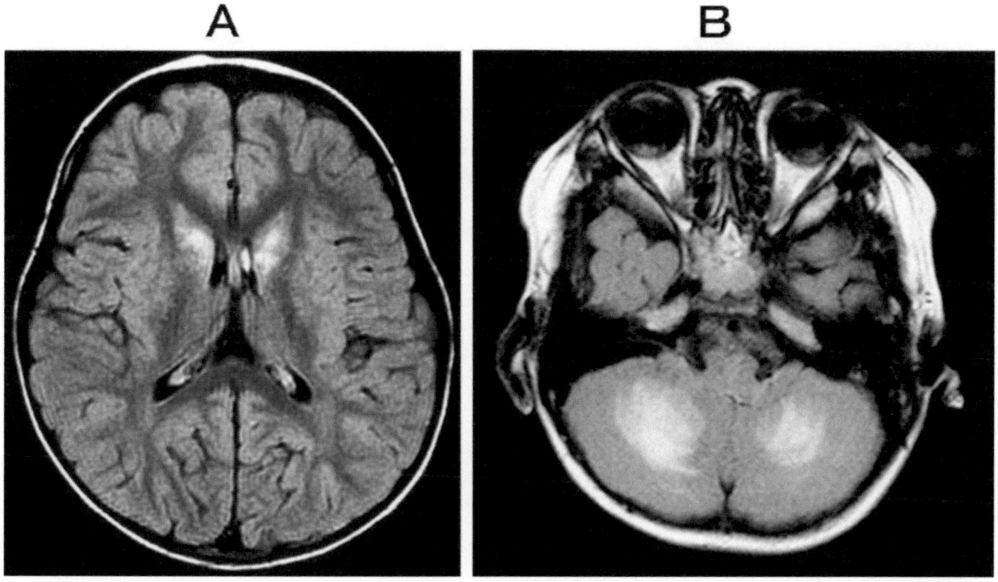

Fig. 3. MRI of patients with neurodegenerative disease after treatment for multifocal LCH show high signals at the basal ganglia (**A:** Flair, TR=9000) and the cerebellar dentate nuclear area (**B:** Flair, TR=9000).

3. Management of LCH-induced CDI

3.1 Definition of CDI response to treatment

Complete response (CR) could be defined as no further need for DDAVP therapy, while partial response (PR) could be defined as a reduction (>50%) in the DDAVP dosage. Although Minehan *et al.* (**27**) included improvement in computed tomography or MRI findings in their evaluation criteria, Grois *et al.* (**7**) concluded that the pituitary stalk thickness changes in a highly variable manner and does not correlate clearly with the treatment outcome.

3.2 Detection of partial CDI

Broadbent *et al.* (**13**) reported that ten of 14 children with LCH-induced CDI had "complete" CDI at onset, while the other four had "partial" CDI. This suggests that, in some cases of LCH, the early phase of CDI can be detected. Such conditions have also been described as partial, transient, or subclinical CDI. In one trial with 21 LCH patients who did not have CDI and had had LCH for less than four years (**11**), when the response of urinary AVP to water deprivation was measured every six months, it was found that 24% had subnormal responses during the initial test and CDI subsequently developed in two. However, it seemed difficult to predict precisely when CDI develops. Notably, Broadbent *et al.* (**13**) also showed that CDI improved transiently during prednisolone therapy in one case and improved permanently after etoposide therapy in another. In addition, Ottaviano *et al.* **(26)** also successfully reversed partial CDI by using 2-chloro-deoxyadenosine (2-CDA). However, preventing the progression from partial CDI to complete CDI by treatment does not seem to be an easy task.

3.3 Irradiation therapy of CDI

LCH-induced CDI has been treated with irradiation with or without systemic chemotherapy **(13, 27-29)**. In the past, hypothalamic-pituitary radiation therapy (HPRT) was the standard treatment for LCH-induced CDI in adults as well as in children **(27)**. According to Minehan *et al.* **(27)**, 36% of their HPRT-treated patients (10/28) responded (22% CR and 14% PR), whereas none in the untreated control group responded. It should be noted that five of the six complete responders were irradiated within 14 days of the diagnosis of CDI, and that three of the five patients (60%) who were treated with more than 15 Gy responded, as compared to seven of 23 patients (30%) who were treated with less than 15 Gy. In addition, eight of the ten responders (80%) were female, whereas 16 of the 35 non-responders (46%) were female. Greenberger **(28)** emphasized that the most important variable in achieving a CR or PR is the speed with which therapy is initiated after the onset of symptoms: it was suggested that therapy should be instituted within 7 days, preferably sooner. However, while these observations indicate the importance and superiority of early intervention with irradiation in CDI, a risk/benefit ratio needs to be determined. In pediatric cases, HPRT is currently not recommended **(30)** and chemotherapy (such as 2-CDA) is preferred to irradiation **(28, 30).** In addition, prolonged low dose systemic chemotherapy is indicated **(30).**

3.4 DDAVP

A synthetic analog of arginine vasopressin is the drug of choice in the treatment of CDI. Nasal or oral administration of DDAVP, a long-acting vasopressin analog, reduces the daily urinary volume (**31**). To maintain normal urinary volume and control the symptoms of CDI, 5–20 μg of nasal DDAVP is required per day. As little as 2.5μg may be sufficient, but the usual dose is 5–15μg/day. In oral DDAVP, the tablet contains 100μg of desmopressin acetate and the maximum plasma concentration after a single oral administration of 100μg DDAVP is obtained at 90 min (**31**). The average oral DDAVP dose required to obtain good control of CDI is about 20 times higher than the intranasal dose. Subcutaneous DDAVP is also available, which is useful for the treatment of infants with CDI and appears to be superior to oral or intranasal DDAVP therapy (**32**). Since the major complication of DDAVP therapy is water intoxication and hyponatremia, careful dose titration is required.

3.5 Optimal measures for APHD and ND disease

Growth hormone deficiency, thyroid dysfunction, and sex hormone (LH/FSH, testosterone) deficiency should be treated by hormonal replacement. In children, growth hormone deficiency is most common, whereas sex hormone deficiency is more frequent in adults. When the disease progresses into panhypopituitarism, cortisol replacement is also required. To date, while several reports have indicated that CDI can be reversed (as discussed above), this has not been observed for APHD (**2,22,23**). There is one exception: Makras *et al.* (**33**) reported that a 35-year-old female resumed normal menstrual cycling after steroid administration. Since the hypothalamic-pituitary space-occupying mass lesions of LCH respond very well to 2-CDA (**2, 26, 34**), additional studies are needed to determine whether early administration of 2-CDA could reverse APHD as well as CDI.

Established ND disease is very difficult to treat. Although several reports have suggested that all-trans retinoic acid or a combination of vincristine/AraC and intravenous high dose gamma-globulin (IVIG) may have some efficacy (**35-37**), it remains unclear whether any specific type of initial systemic chemotherapy for multifocal LCH patients can limit the later occurrence of ND disease (**38**). There is an urgent need for research that can identify an innovative therapy for such cases.

4. CDI and other CNS complications experienced in the Japanese LCH study

The cases of CDI, APHD and ND disease were analyzed in the cohort of patients treated with the JLSG-96/-02 protocols from 1996 to 2009 in Japan (**39**). CDI was detected in 12.4% (43/348) of pediatric multifocal LCH patients with a median follow-up of 5.0 (range, 0.2–14.0) years, with the shortest follow-up of alive patients being 0.8 years from the initiation of treatment. Of these 43 cases, CDI was detected before LCH diagnosis in 13 cases, at the LCH diagnosis in 12 cases, during the induction/maintenance treatment in five cases, and after off therapy at a median of 21 months (range, 4–116) in the remaining 12 cases. The incidence of CDI after the initiation therapy was 5.6% in our JLSG protocols, which is lower than 9.3% by Grois et al. (5). Data indicate that our treatment protocol effectively reduces the incidence of CDI by preventing the new occurrence. Of the 43 CDI patients, APHD was noted in 30.2% (13/43), with growth hormone deficiency being observed in ten of these patients. Six patients developed ND disease. In total, chemotherapy completely resolved CDI in two patients, which suggests that early intervention with chemotherapy may be able to reverse CDI (**39**).

5. Recommendations and future trials

In practice, when LCH patients, particularly those with craniofacial bone lesions, are diagnosed, treated and followed up, they must be examined carefully for any signs suggesting that CDI is developing. In particular, inquiring about the symptoms of polydipsia/polyuria and occasional tests for plasma osmolarity with plasma AVP may help to diagnose CDI early after onset. Moreover, in young females, the presence of amenorrhea and/or morbid obesity could be a first sign of pituitary dysfunction together with CDI. Repeated brain MRI examinations are also useful for detecting the early signs of CDI and/or ND disease. Once the precise diagnosis of CDI has been made, nasal or oral DDAVP is a safe therapeutic option that effectively controls CDI. Patients with anterior pituitary dysfunction require other hormonal replacement therapies.

Effective measures that can reverse CDI or other CDI-related neurological complications, or prevent them from newly occurring, remain elusive. Studies have shown that in LCH-induced CDI cases, the CDI is already present at the start of chemotherapy in half of the cases, while the remaining half develop CDI during chemotherapy or after off therapy. Ideally, the early introduction of chemotherapy should be able to reverse pre-existing CDI and prevent the new occurrence of CDI. Unfortunately, however, therapeutic regimens for patients with LCH that consistently achieve these goals have not yet been identified. However, we recently found that IVIG may be able to prevent the progression of ND disease in patients with LCH **(10, 35)**. Given this observation and the fact that IVIG is also effective for other CNS inflammatory diseases, we have hypothesized that pre-emptive measures that include high dose IVIG may reduce the incidence of LCH-related CNS diseases, namely CDI and its related neurological complications, if they are given early and are combined with chemotherapy. To that end, we have proposed that the initial treatment of patients with "CNS-risk"-LCH should contain a high dose (2g/kg/dose) of IVIG combined with conventional induction chemotherapy (**40**). However, precise efficacy of immunomodulatory agents such as IVIG for treating LCH, particularly for preventing the development of LCH-related CNS diseases, needs to be explored by future studies.

6. References

[1] Maghnie M, Cosi G, Genovese E, et al. Central diabetes insipidus in children and young adults.N Engl J Med 2000;343:998-1007.

[2] Adam Z, Balsíková K, Krejcí M, et al.Central diabetes insipidus in adult patients--the first sign of Langerhans cell histiocytosis and Erdheim-Chester disease. Three case studies and literature review.Vnitr Lek.2010; 56:138-148.

[3] Grois N, Fahrner B, Arceci RJ, et al. Central nervous system disease in Langerhans cell histiocytosis. J Pediatr.2010;156:873-881.

[4] Abla O, Egeler RM, Weitzman S. Langerhans cell histiocytosis: Current concepts and treatments. Cancer Treat Rev. 2010; 36:354-359.

[5] Grois N, Pötschger U, Prosch H, et al. Risk factors for diabetes insipidus in Langerhans cell histiocytosis. Pediatr Blood Cancer 2006; 46: 228-233.

[6] Leger J, Velasquez A, Garel C, et al. Thickened pituitary stalk on magnetic resonance imaging in children with central diabetes insipidus. J Clin Endocrinol Metab.1999; 84:1954-1960.

[7] Grois N, Prayer D, Prosch H, et al. Course and clinical impact of magnetic resonance imaging findings in diabetes insipidus associated with Langerhans cell histiocytosis. Pediatr Blood Cancer 2004;43:59-65.

[8] Lee MH, Choi HY, Sung YA, Lee JK.High signal intensity of the posterior pituitary gland on T1-weighted MR images. Correlation with plasma vasopressin concentration to water deprivation. ActaRadiol. 2001; 42:129-134.

[9] Wnorowski M, Prosch H, Prayer D, et al. Pattern and course of neurodegeneration in Langerhans cell histiocytosis. J Pediatr 2008; 153:127–132

[10] Imashuku S, Shioda Y, Kobayashi R, et al. Neurodegenerative central nervous system disease as late sequelae of Langerhans cell histiocytosis. Report from the Japan LCH Study Group.Haematologica.2008; 93:615-618.

[11] Dunger DB, Broadbent V, Yeoman E, et al. The frequency and natural history of diabetes insipidus in children with Langerhans cell histiocytosis. N Engl J Med 1989; 321:1157-1162.

[12] Imashuku S, Kinugawa N, Matsuzaki A, et al. Langerhans cell histiocytosis with multifocal bone lesions: comparative clinical features between single and multi-systems.Int J Hematol 2009; 90:506-512.

[13] Broadbent V, Pritchard J. Diabetes insipidus associated with Langerhans cell histiocytosis: is it reversible? Med Pediatr Oncol 1997;28: 289-293.

[14] Matoussi N, Aissa K, Fitouri Z, et al. Central diabetes insipidus: diagnostic difficulties. Ann Endocrinol (Paris).2008 ;69:231-239.

[15] Donadieu J, Egeler RM, Pritchard J. Langerhans cell histiocytosis: a clinical update. In (Edit by Weitzman and Egeler RM) Histiocytic Disorders of Children and Adults; Basic Science, Clinical Features and Therapy (Cambridge University Press 2005), pp95-129
[16] Schmitt S, Wichmann W, Martin E, et al. Pituitary stalk thickening with diabetes insipidus preceding typical manifestations of Langerhans cell histiocytosis in children. Eur J Pediatr.1993;152:399-401.
[17] Prosch H, Grois N, Bökkerink J, et al. Central diabetes insipidus: Is it Langerhans cell histiocytosis of the pituitary stalk? A diagnostic pitfall. Pediatr Blood Cancer 2006; 46:363-366
[18] Conley A, Manjila S, Guan H, et al. Non-Langerhans cell histiocytosis with isolated CNS involvement: An unusual variant of Erdheim-Chester disease. Neuropathology. 2010; 30: 634-647
[19] Abe T. Lymphocytic infundibulo- neurohypophysitis and infundibulo-panhypophysitis regarded as lymphocytic hypophysitis variant. Brain Tumor Pathol.2008; 25: 59-66.
[20] Arslan A, Karaarslan E, Dincer A.High intensity signal of the posterior pituitary. A study with horizontal direction of frequency-encoding and fat suppression MR techniques.ActaRadiol.1999; 40:142-145.
[21] Lin KD, Lin JD, Hsu HH, et al. Endocrinological aspects of Langerhans cell histiocytosis complicated with diabetes insipidus. J Endocrinol Invest.1998;21:428-433.
[22] Modan-Moses D, Weintraub M, Meyerovitch J, et al. Hypopituitarism in Langerhans cell histiocytosis: seven cases and literature review. J Endocrinol Invest.2001; 24: 612-617.
[23] Kaltsas, GA,Powles TB, Evanson J, et al. Hypothalamo-pituitary abnormalities in adult patients with Langerhans cell histiocytosis: clinical, endocrinological, and radiological features and response to treatment. J ClinEndocrinolMetab 2000; 85: 1370-1376
[24] Amato MC, Elias LL, Elias J, et al. Endocrine disorders in pediatric - onset Langerhans Cell Histiocytosis. Horm Metab Res 2006; 38: 746-751
[25] Donadieu J, Rolon MA, Pion I, et al. Incidence of growth hormone deficiency in pediatric-onset Langerhans cell histiocytosis: Efficacy and safety of growth hormone treatment. J Clin Endocrinol Metab 2004; 89:604–609.
[26] Ottaviano F, Finlay JL. Diabetes insipidus and Langerhans cell histiocytosis: a case report of reversibility with 2-chlorodeoxyadenosine. J Pediatr Hematol Oncol. 2003;25: 575-577.
[27] Minehan KJ, Chen MG, Zimmerman D, et al. Radiation therapy for diabetes insipidus caused by Langerhans cell histiocytosis. Int J Radiat Oncol Biol Phys. 1992; 23: 519-524.
[28] Greenberger JS. Radiation therapy in children continued need to assess risk versus gain. Int J Radiat Oncol Biol Phys. 1992; 23: 675-676.
[29] Rosenzweig KE, Arceci RJ, Tarbell NJ.Diabetes insipidus secondary to Langerhans' cell histiocytosis: is radiation therapy indicated? Med Pediatr Oncol 1997; 29:36-40.
[30] Abla O, Weitzman S, Minkov M, et al. Diabetes insipidus in Langerhans cell histiocytosis: When is treatment indicated? Pediatr Blood Cancer 2009; 52:555-556.

[31] Fukuda I, Hizuka N, Takano K.Oral DDAVP is a good alternative therapy for patients with central diabetes insipidus: experience of five-year treatment. Endocr J. 2003; 50: 437-443.

[32] Rivkees SA, Dunbar N, Wilson TA. The management of central diabetes insipidus in infancy: desmopressin, low renal solute load formula, thiazide diuretics. J Pediatr Endocrinol Metab 2007;20:459-469.

[33] Makras P, Papadogias D, Kontogeorgos G, et al. Spontaneous gonadotrophin deficiency recovery in an adult patient with Langerhans cell histiocytosis (LCH).Pituitary2005;8:169-174.

[34] Dhall G, Finlay JL, Dunkel IJ, et al. Analysis of outcome for patients with mass lesions of the central nervous system due to Langerhans cell histiocytosis treated with 2-chlorodeoxyadenosine. Pediatr Blood Cancer 2008; 50:72-79.

[35] Imashuku S Treatment of Neurodegenerative CNS Disease in Langerhans Cell Histiocytosis, with a Combination of Intravenous Immunoglobulin and Chemotherapy. Pediatr Blood Cancer 2008;50:308–311

[36] Idbaih A, Donadieu J, Barthez, MA, et al. Retinoic Acid Therapy in ''Degenerative-Like'' Neuro-Langerhans Cell Histiocytosis: A Prospective Pilot Study. Pediatr Blood Cancer 2004; 43:55–58

[37] Allen CE, Flores R, Rauch R, et al. Neurodegenerative central nervous system Langerhans cell histiocytosis and coincident hydrocephalus treated with vincristine/cytosine arabinoside. Pediatr Blood Cancer 2010;54:416–423.

[38] Imashuku S, Okazaki NA, Nakayama M, et al.VCR/AraC Chemotherapy and ND-CNS-LCH. Pediatr Blood Cancer 2008; 50: 308-311.

[39] ShiodaY, Adachi S, Imashuku S, et al. Analysis of 43 cases of Langerhans cell histiocytosis (LCH)- induced central diabetes insipidus registered in the JLSG-96 and JLSG -02 studies in Japan (in preparation)

[40] Imashuku S. High dose immunoglobulin (IVIG) may reduce the incidence of Langerhans cell histiocytosis (LCH)-associated central nervous system involvement.CNS Neurol Disord Drug Targets.2009; 8:380-386.

2

Diabetes Insipidus and Traumatic Brain Injury

Yi-Chun Chou, Tzu-Yuan Wang and Li-Wei Chou
China Medical University Hospital,
Department of Physical Medicine and Rehabilitation
Taiwan, R.O.C.

1. Introduction

Traumatic brain injury (TBI) is a leading cause of mortality and morbidity worldwide and is the major cause of disability among children and young adults in the United States (1999; Adekoya, Thurman et al. 2002). Recent data show that there are over a million emergency room visits for TBI in the United States annually. The majority of such emergency room visits are for patients with mild TBI, defined as a post-resuscitation Glasgow Coma Scale with a score of 13–15 (Teasdale and Jennett 1974). However, approximately 300,000 TBI victims are hospitalized annually. Of these, over 50,000 die and over half of the survivors have permanent neurobehavioral and quality of life problems, the most common being memory and concentration deficits, depression, anxiety, fatigue, and loss of emotional well-being (Levin, Gary et al. 1990; Kraus and McArthur 1996; Hellawell, Taylor et al. 1999; Kelly, McArthur et al. 2006; Rutland-Brown, Langlois et al. 2006).

Diabetes insipidus (DI) from post-TBI hypopituitarism was first reported in 1921 (Rouvillois, Reverchon et al. 1921) and, in the 1970s, multiple case reports were published, documenting posterior pituitary dysfunction (Massol, Humbert et al. 1987; Halimi, Sigal et al. 1988). DI may be of a central (neurogenic), nephrogenic, gestational, dipsogenic, adipsic, or psychogenic type. The most common DI, the central type, which follows brain injury or surgery to the region of the pituitary and hypothalamus, is noted in previous literature review. DI is characterized by a diminished secretion of antidiuretic hormone, also known as arginine vasopressin (AVP). Neuroendocrine abnormalities following brain injury may occur with a much higher prevalence than previously realized, and represent an underdiagnosed consequence of brain injury.

The prevalence of central DI among all kinds of neuroendocrine derangements after TBI in acute to chronic phases was 1.7%-26%. The development of DI seems to correlate with the severity of trauma in spite of more cases of permanent DI being reported in mild TBI cases. Central DI caused by brain injury is detectable because of polyuria and polydipsia in patients, but the occasions of DI are almost transient, leading to ignorance of its precise diagnosis and adequate treatment.

In this chapter, diabetes insipidus was considered as central diabetes insipidus, which is a result of TBI.

2. Epidemiology of diabetes insipidus after traumatic brain injury

TBI involves, not only the primary mechanical event, but also secondary implications, such as pituitary insufficiency. Large neuropathological studies, including a total of 638 cases,

established a large frequency of 26.4% to 86% hypothalamic-pituitary damage in patients who died as a consequence of head injury (Ceballos 1966; Kornblum and Fisher 1969; Crompton 1971; Pierucci, Gherson et al. 1971; Harper, Doyle et al. 1986; Salehi, Kovacs et al. 2007). Schneider et al. (Schneider, Kreitschmann-Andermahr et al. 2007) conducted 19 studies, which included 1137 patients, and pointed out that the pooled prevalence of hypopituitarism in the chronic phase after TBI was 27.5% (95% confidence interval [CI], 22.8%-28.9%). The prevalence of DI ranged 1.7% to 26% among all kinds of neuroendocrine derangements after brain injury in acute to chronic phases (Klose, Juul et al. 2007; Behan, Phillips et al. 2008). In a prospective cross-sectional and longitudinal study on posterior pituitary function after TBI, the prevalence of DI, diagnosed using the water deprivation test criterion standard, was 26% in the acute phase (Agha, Sherlock et al. 2005) and 6.9% among long-term survivors (Agha, Thornton et al. 2004).
Literature regarding adults diagnosed with DI following TBI have flourished since 1998, and the findings of key studies are summarized in Table 1. Some observations are supported by a series of recent findings reported by Agha et al. In the study of 102 TBI survivors assessed at a median of 17 months following moderate to severe injury, acute DI and permanent DI were detected in 21.6% and 6.9% of patients, respectively. In 2003, Agha and colleagues also discovered a high frequency of DI (26%) in survivors (n=50) of moderate to severe TBI (range of 7-12 days).

Study period	Author, year	Number	Population	Onset Time of DI after TBI	Severity of TBI (GCS)	Prevalence of DI
-	Boughey et al, 2004 (Boughey, Yost et al. 2004)	888	USA	176 days	<6	2.9%
1998–2002	Alfonso Leal-Cerro, 2005 (Leal-Cerro, Flores et al. 2005)	170	Male: 88% Mean age 28 years Spain	Episode of TBI	<8: 100%	1.7%
2000-2002	Agha et al, 2004 (Agha, Thornton et al. 2004)	102	Males:83% 15-65 years Ireland	range 6–36 months, Median 17 months	9–12: 44% <9: 56%	Acute DI: 21.6% Permanent DI: 6.9%
2003	Agha et al, 2004 (Agha, Rogers et al. 2004)	50	Male: 76 %,Age:- Ireland	12 days (range 7–20)	9–12: 36% <9: 64%	26%
2003-2005	Klose et al, 2007 (Klose, Juul et al. 2007)	104	Male: 75% median age 41 (range 18–64) years Denmark	13 (10–27) months postinjury	13–15: 42% 9–12: 19% <9: 38%	2%
2003	Aimaretti et al, 2004 (Aimaretti, Ambrosio et al. 2004)	100	Male 69% age 37.1±1.8 years Italian	3 months	13–15: 55% 9–12: 24% <9: 21%	4%

Table 1. Prevalence of diabetes insipidus after trauamtic brain injury across countries

2.1 Mechanism of diabetes insipidus after traumatic brain injury

DI is characterized by a diminished release of AVP, resulting in variable degrees of hypotonic polyuria. Paucity of AVP may be caused by disorders that act at one or more of the sites involved in AVP secretion, namely, the hypothalamic osmoreceptors; the supraoptic or paraventricular nuclei; or the superior portion of the supraopticohypophyseal tract (Rose, Narins et al. 2001) (Fig. 1). Autopsy results have demonstrated different types of lesions, from damage to the pituitary capsule (the most frequent form of pituitary damage after TBI, occurring in 23.3%-59% of patients) to injury to the anterior and the posterior lobes and the pituitary stalk, in the form of hemorrhage, necrosis, and fibrosis (Ceballos 1966; Kornblum and Fisher 1969; Crompton 1971; Pierucci, Gherson et al. 1971; Harper, Doyle et al. 1986; Salehi, Kovacs et al. 2007). In contrast, damage to the tract below the median eminence or to the posterior pituitary generally induces only transient polyuria because AVP produced in the hypothalamus can still be secreted into the systemic circulation via the portal capillaries in the median eminence (Rose, Narins et al. 2001). Therefore, the severity of injury is unlikely to be the cause of hypopituitarism that would more likely be determined as trauma characteristics and/or unknown vascular mechanisms (Aimaretti, Ambrosio et al. 2004). There has ever been a report, showing that DI occurred secondary to penetrating spinal cord trauma (Kuzeyli, Cakir et al. 2001).

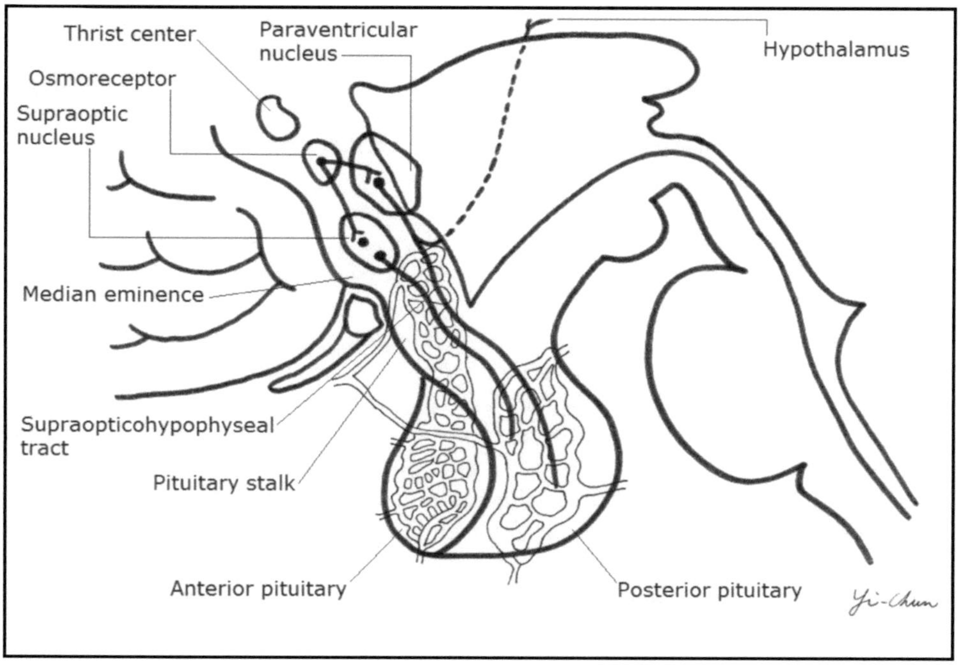

Fig. 1. Arginine vasopressin is transported from the hypothalamus through the neural component of the pituitary stalk and stored in nerve terminals in the posterior pituitary.

2.1.1 Imaging studies of the hypothalamic-pituitary region after traumatic brain injuy

The posterior pituitary is known to be hyperintense on sagittal T1-weighted magnetic resonance imaging (MRI) of normal subjects. The absence of this finding serves as a nonspecific indicator of DI, although the frequency of hyperintensity declines with aging in normal subjects (Brooks, el Gammal et al. 1989). The frequency of these radiologic abnormalities in patients with DI is poorly defined. Maghnie et al. (Maghnie, Cosi et al. 2000) investigated the clinical presentation, the morphologic characteristics of the pituitary region on MRI, and the size of the pituitary stalk over time in patients who had DI from a variety of causes. The initial radiological findings, based on Marshall Classification, and/or the presence of cranial fractures did not predict the development of hypopituitarism (Bondanelli, De Marinis et al. 2004).

With regard to the anatomical integrity of the hypothalamic-pituitary region, autopsy series from patients with fatal TBI displayed different degrees of damage to this region (Kornblum and Fisher 1969; Lieberman, Oberoi et al. 2001). This further supports the hypothesis that TBI severity is an important risk factor in the development of hypopituitarism. However, in the study made by Bondanelli et al. (Bondanelli, De Marinis et al. 2004), a significant number of patients with minimal TBI exhibited some degree of hypopituitarism. Also, in the Bondanelli study, the occurrence of anatomical lesions on MRI was low in patients with severe TBI and hypopituitarism. This was also seen in the series of studies made by Cytowic et al. (Cytowic, Smith et al. 1986). Therefore, in patients without radiological alteration, the functional damage to the hypothalamic-pituitary region may be due to a secondary hypoxic insult. Another possibility is diffused axonal injury caused by the acceleration-deceleration along rotational forces in motor vehicle crashes. Diffused axonal injury is the principal pathology in 40 to 50 percent of TBI hospital admissions, and is the predominant cause of loss of consciousness. Secondary to shearing injury, diffused axonal injury is seen in the midline structures. Most often, the initial CT and MRI scans have no specific findings and, therefore, it is only conclusively diagnosed microscopically (Cytowic, Smith et al. 1986). This explains why some patients with TBI, who undergo radiological scans, do not display any specific findings.

However, recent MRI studies of the pituitary demonstrated pathological changes consistent with vascular injury. In the acute phase, the pituitary glands of TBI patients are significantly enlarged as compared with normal healthy control subjects. Many also demonstrate other abnormalities, such as hemorrhage, infarction, signal abnormalities, and/or partial stalk transection (Maiya, Newcombe et al. 2008). In the chronic phase, patients often demonstrate pituitary volume loss or empty sella, followed by abnormal pituitary gland signal heterogeneity, perfusion deficits, and/or lack of posterior pituitary signal (Schneider, Samann et al. 2007). The recently published study of 70 TBI patients with long-term follow-up suggests that the degree of brain injury, as defined by acute CT (presence of diffused brain swelling and evacuated intracerebral hematoma or multiple contusions, in particular), is the strongest predictor of subsequent hypopituitarism (Bavisetty, McArthur et al. 2008).

2.2 Differential diagnosis of diabetes insipidus following traumatic brain injury after neurosurgery

Polyuria can be defined as a urine output exceeding 3 L/24 h in adults and 2 L/m2 in children. It must be differentiated from the more common complaints of frequency or nocturia, which are not associated with an increase in the total urine output. Differential diagnosis has to be kept in mind when TBI patients undergoing neurosurgery have huge amounts of urine output because most cases of polyuria, at this time, are not caused by DI (Seckl and Dunger 1989). The more common causes are excretion of excess fluid administered during surgery and an osmotic diuresis, resulting from treatment aimed at minimizing cerebral edema using mannitol or glucocorticoids (Bohn, Davids et al. 2005).

The diagnosis of DI following TBI in the immediate postoperative period may be more difficult because polyuria can occur during this period, secondary to a variety of causes. When polyuria begins, establish whether it is secondary to water or solute excretion. A solute diuresis may be a result of hyperglycemia; inability to retain sodium, secondary to corticosteroid deficiency; high urea levels; or the residual effect of osmotic diuretics so commonly used in neurosurgical procedures. When the diuresis is secondary to solute excretion, the urinary specific gravity is usually between 1.009 and 1.035; the urine osmolality is usually between 250 and 320 mOsm/kg; the serum sodium is normal or slightly decreased; and thirst is not usually a complaint. When the diuresis is secondary to water excretion, the urinary specific gravity is usually between 1.001 and 1.005; the urine osmolality is between 50 and 150 mOsm/kg; the serum sodium is usually normal or increased; and thirst is usually a prominent feature. The latter picture is, of course, what is seen in diabetes insipidus.

When it is determined that the diuresis is secondary to the excretion of a water load, the differential diagnosis includes the following:

1. Diabetes insipidus.
2. Chronic renal insufficiency. Renal function tests are abnormal and the patient is usually azotemic.
3. Multiple myeloma, amyloidosis, sickle cell disease, and a peculiar phenomenon sometimes seen after relief of obstructive uropathy are rarer causes of an inability to concentrate urine. These problems usually cause little difficulty in the differential diagnosis.
4. Recovery phase of acute tubular necrosis. The clinical sequence of events in this problem usually makes the diagnosis clear.
5. Fluid overload. Careful attention must be paid to fluid administration during the intraoperative and the immediate postoperative periods when the patient may receive excessive amounts of parenteral fluids. If these fluids are electrolyte-free and do not cause a solute diuresis, the patient may retain excessive quantities of water. As the patient excretes this excessive water load, he may have an output which exceeds his intake. These conditions can be differentiated from DI by measuring urine osmolality, the response to water restriction, and the administration of AVP.

You may conclude that a patient has DI if either

1. The plasma sodium exceeds 150 mmol/ l in the presence of polyuria of > 3 L /24 h in an acute clinical setting; or
2. Following an overnight water deprivation test or an 8-h observed water deprivation test, urine osmolality is less than 600 mOsmol/kg; or
3. Considering a hypertonic saline water infusion test with measuring plasma AVP level while water deprivation test as a great burden to patients;
4. If these do not occur, responsiveness of the renal tubule should be demonstrated by vasopressin administration.

Once DI after TBI is adequately evaluated and accurately measured, the replacement of AVP may be considered.

3. Outcome and association factors of diabetes insipidus after traumatic brain injury

Admittedly, the pathophysiology of TBI is complex and is still poorly understood in many ways because there is a wide spectrum of injury severity, injury mechanisms, and brain injury patterns across all age ranges. In spite of more cases of permanent DI being reported in mild head injury cases (Segal-Lieberman, Karasik et al. 2000; Chou, Wang et al. 2009), the development of DI seems to correlate with the severity of trauma (Tsagarakis, Tzanela et al. 2005). The pooled prevalence of hypopituitarism is greater in patients with severe TBI compared with those with mild or moderate TBI (Klose, Juul et al. 2007; Salehi, Kovacs et al. 2007; Hadjizacharia, Beale et al. 2008). Recent prospective data suggest that the incidence of DI may be as high as 26% in the acute phase immediately following TBI, although up to 70% of cases fully recover from DI within 12 months (Agha, Sherlock et al. 2005). The incidence of acute DI in severe TBI is high, especially in penetrating injuries (Hadjizacharia, Beale et al. 2008). Independent risk factors for DI include a Glasgow Coma Scale lower or equal to 8, cerebral edema, and a head Abbreviated Injury Score higher than 3 (Hadjizacharia, Beale et al. 2008). The risk of pituitary insufficiency increases in patients with severe TBI as opposed to those with mild TBI [odds ratio (OR) 10.1, 95% confidence interval (CI) 2.1-48.4, P = 0.004], and in those patients with increased intracerebral pressure (OR 6.5, 95% CI 1.0-42.2, P = 0.03) (Klose, Juul et al. 2007). Posttraumatic DI was not associated with the presence of anterior hypopituitarism but was associated with more severe head trauma and the presence of cerebral edema on CT scan (Agha, Thornton et al. 2004). Moreover, severe TBI associated with basilar skull fracture, hypothalamic edema, prolonged unresponsiveness, hyponatremia, and/or hypotension is associated with a higher occurrence of endocrinopathy (Powner, Boccalandro et al. 2006).

By contrast, Agha et al. reported in 2003 that the occurrence of post-trauma DI is unrelated to the severity of TBI, as assessed by the Glasgow Coma Scale score. Lieberman et al. (Lieberman, Oberoi et al. 2001) also found no correlation between severity of head injury and pituitary dysfunction. Trauma severity was not uniformly identified as predictive of post-traumatic DI, which may be explained by a variety of reasons. The choice of diagnostic criteria, timing after TBI, identification of TBI severity, and thus of tests and cut-off limits, as well as that of inclusion and exclusion criteria, are of paramount importance in prevalence studies and the identification of predictors. For example, DI has been reported to occur in 13% of patients in the late head injury period, with diagnosis made on the basis of random plasma and urine osmolalities, which are insufficiently accurate for either clinical or research purposes (Bohnen, Twijnstra et al. 1993). Also, alcohol and drug intoxication are serious confounders of the initial GCS scoring. Not all studies exclude patients with chronic alcohol or drug abuse and, as a result, this obvious confounder may have contributed to the observed inequalities.

DI from post-traumatic hypopituitarism had been documented as a potential contributor to morbidity and, possibly, mortality. Boughey et al. (Boughey, Yost et al. 2004) reported that patients who develop DI early (in the first 3 days) have a higher mortality rate than those who develop DI later. The mean onset time of DI in nonsurvivors (1.5+-0.7 days) is shorter compared with survivors (8.9+-10.2 days) (P<0.001). The developement of DI after TBI carries a 69% mortality rate, and if the onset is within the first 3 days after injury, the mortality rate rises to 86%.

3.1 Transient or persistent diabetes insipidus

Actually, destruction of the hypothalamic centers or division of the supraoptic tract above the median eminence causes permanent DI. Transection below the median eminence, even removal of the posterior pituitary lobe, produces only a transient polyuria. However, DI, following brain injury or surgery in the hypothalamic-pituitary area, can follow a variety of patterns in its development. Early prognostication as regards the permanence of DI should not be made because of a marked variation in the eventual outcome. Cerebral edema generally appears within 12 to 24 hours and is most marked at 48 to 72 hours. This edema may functionally impair cells which are structurally intact. A temporary DI can develop and is subsequently resolved as the edema clears. There are varying degrees of chronic antidiuretic hormone deficiency, with the urinary output being related to the number of viable cells.

These initial insults, as well as transient events and treatments during the early injury phase, can evidently impact hypothalamic-pituitary function both acutely and chronically after injury. In most occasions, DI is transient, but persisting DI may develop with an incidence of 6.9%-7.5% among TBI victims (Tsagarakis, Tzanela et al. 2005). Severe damage to the hypothalamus or the supraopticohypophyseal tract by neurosurgery or trauma often results in a typical triphasic response (Rose, Narins et al. 2001; Ghirardello, Hopper et al. 2006) (Fig. 2). There is an initial polyuric phase, beginning within 24 hours and lasting 4 to 5 days. This phase reflects the inhibition of AVP release because of hypothalamic dysfunction (Seckl and Dunger 1989). This is followed, on days 6 to 11, by an antidiuretic phase, in which stored hormone is slowly released from the degenerating posterior pituitary. During this stage, excessive water intake can lead to hyponatremia in a manner similar to that in the syndrome of inappropriate AVP secretion. Permanent DI may then ensue after the posterior pituitary stores are depleted.

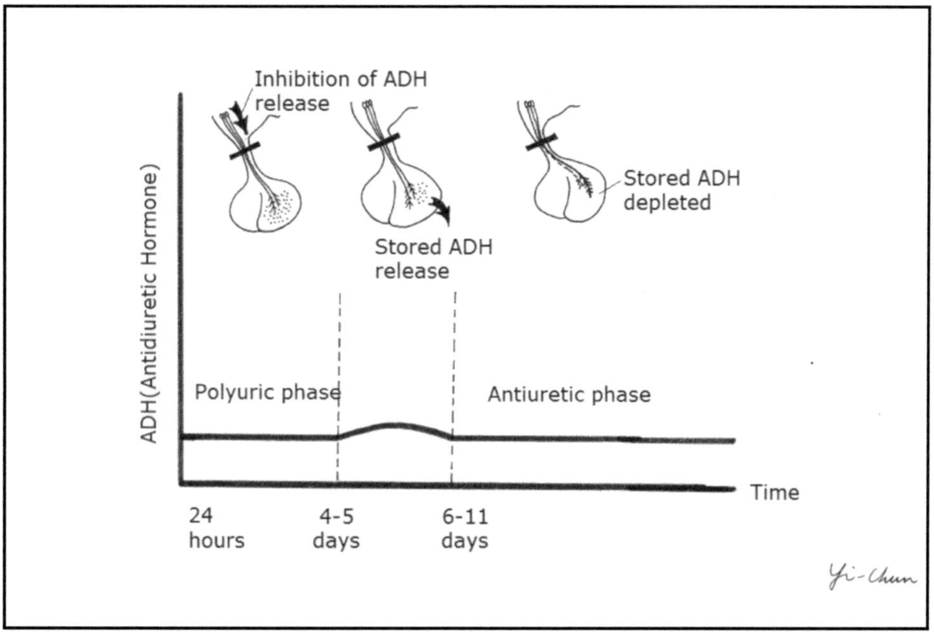

Fig. 2. Tri-phases of central diabetes insipidus after severe damage to the hypothalamus or supraopticohypophyseal tract

There was rarely any statement or discussion associated with the factors implicated in the persistence and the duration of post-trauma DI. Although one study has discovered that postoperative hypernatremia (higher than 145 mmol/L) within the first five days has a high predictor value for permanent DI development (Sigounas, Sharpless et al. 2008). Different phases of post-head injury were presented with various amounts of urine output clinically. Post-traumatic DI is often transient, and suggests that patients need to be followed up to determine the true prevalence of late DI following TBI (Edwards and Clark 1986).

4. Management of diabetes insipidus after traumatic brain injury

The probability of developing hypopituitarism is based on the severity of the TBI. However, discrepancies in recent studies indicate that minimal TBI can also result in hypopituitarism. Thus, patients with moderate to severe TBI must be screened, and those with minimal TBI must be monitored for hypopituitarism. Alterations in pituitary hormones may develop subtly or generate clinical manifestations similar to those attributed to head trauma. Therefore, pituitary dysfunction may be overlooked or viewed as a result of postconcussional causes and escape diagnosis (Edwards and Clark 1986; Benvenga, Campenni et al. 2000). The modern therapeutic paradigm for moderate and severe TBI victims is centered on the concepts of rapidly treating the primary brain injury, correcting or avoiding secondary brain insults, and optimizing cerebral blood flow and metabolism (Edwards and Clark 1986; Benvenga, Campenni et al. 2000; Kelly, Gonzalo et al. 2000; Agha, Rogers et al. 2004; Dimopoulou, Tsagarakis et al. 2004). The temporal relationship between TBI and the occurrence of hypopituitarism is observed in three phases, namely, acute, recovery, and chronic. Agha et al. examined the prevalence of anterior and posterior pituitary dysfunctions in the acute (7–21 days) phase following TBI, and those series-identified deficiencies in need of immediate replacement, such as ACTH deficiency and posterior pituitary dysfunction (Agha, Rogers et al. 2004).

Adequate secretion of AVP is crucial in water homeostasis. Inadequate AVP secretion leads to varying degrees of water loss. Water intake may be inadequate to compensate for the water loss because of impaired cognition, physical disability, or coexistent hypodipsia that may occur in the early post-TBI period. This may lead to hypernatraemic dehydration with increased morbidity and impairment of recovery (Maggiore, Picetti et al. 2009). Therefore, daily sodium measurements and fluid charts are indicated in all TBI patients during the early post-injury period. Therapeutic intervention with desmopressin is indicated in patients with severe forms of this disorder. Caution is required for the occasional development of the syndrome involving inappropriate AVP release that may also occur as a result of brain trauma, and increase the likelihood of seizures. If polyuria persists during the late-phase of TBI, a persistent DI should be appropriately diagnosed and treated.

4.1 Drugs for diabetes insipidus after traumatic brain injury

Considering that the primary problem in DI is the deficient secretion of AVP, control of the polyuria can be achieved by hormone replacement. In the past, intramuscular injections of vasopressin (Pitressin) tannate in oil was used to control, which is no longer available. This preparation had two problems, namely, the requirement of intramuscular administration and the occasional development of antivasopressin antibodies, with a secondary increase in urine output that appear AVP resistant (Vokes, Gaskill et al. 1988). Pitressin has many side effects of anaphylaxis (cardiac arrest and/or shock), circumoral pallor, arrhythmias, decreased cardiac output, angina, myocardial ischemia, peripheral vasoconstriction, gangrene, abdominal cramps, nausea, vomiting, passage of gas, tremor, vertigo, pounding in head, bronchial constriction, sweating, urticaris, cutaneous gangrene et al. Otherwise, pitressin has two actions with V1 and V2 receptors. As DI is caused by decreased V2 receptor function owing to paucity of AVP secretion, it is better to have V2 receptor action alone without V1 receptor action as drug. Consequently, using DDAVP (desmopressin acetate) instead of Pitressin is better. Desmopressin comes in liquid form. That is, it is usually administered intranasally and in an oral tablet form. The usual daily maintenance dose is 10 to 20 µg once or twice a day.

An oral tablet preparation of desmopressin is also available (Stenberg and Lackgren 1994). The absorption of desmopressin in normal persons is decreased by 40 to 50 percent when taken with meals (Rittig, Jensen et al. 1998). The oral form has about one-tenth to one-twentieth the potency of the nasal form because only about five percent is absorbed from the gut. Thus, a 0.1 mg tablet is the equivalent of 2.5 to 5 µg of the nasal spray. Although patients generally prefer the oral preparation because of ease of administration, not all patients have an adequate response. As a result, we recommend starting with the intranasal preparation. This ensures that the patient understands what constitutes a good antidiuretic response prior to performing a trial of oral therapy. If DDAVP cannot be administered intranasally or orally, it can be given subcutaneously. A usual antidiuretic dose is 1 µg, administered subcutaneously every 12 hours. Alternatively, in patients with decreased subcutaneous absorption, 2 µg of desmopressin acetate is given intravenously over one minute, and the duration of action, as judged by increased urine osmolality, is 12 hours or more (Rembratt, Graugaard-Jensen et al. 2004). DDAVP is safe for both the mother and the fetus when administered during pregnancy (Ray 1998).

For the vast majority of patients with DI, desmopressin is readily available, safe, and effective. Nevertheless, with partial DI and/or if the amount of available desmopressin is limited (Thurman, Halterman et al. 2003), the addition of other drugs that increase AVP release, enhance AVP effect on the kidneys (both of which require at least some endogenous AVP secretion), or directly decrease the urine output independent of AVP is rarely necessary. However, these agents, such as chlorpropamide, carbamazepine, clofibrate, thiazide diuretics, or NSAID, are less effective and associated with more adverse effects than desmopressin.

5. Conclusion

DI from post-traumatic hypopituitarism is documented as a potential contributor to morbidity and, possibly, mortality. As the above discussion shows, we suggest and note that

1. Greater awareness of these possible complications of TBI and appropriate testing are encouraged.
2. Assessment of the integrity of AVP secretion, and hypothalamic-pituitary axis is crucial to ensure the survival and the optimal rehabilitation of TBI patients.
3. Physicians should also present clinical symptoms of anterior or posterior pituitary dysfunction, not only for patients with severe TBI who need to be screened, but also for patients with minimal brain injury (Estes and Urban 2005).
4. The identification and the appropriate timely management of hormone deficiencies, such as the replacement and supplementation of desmopressin, are crucial to optimize patient recovery from brain injury, improve quality of life, and avoid long-term adverse outcomes of untreated hypopituitarism.
5. By monitoring pituitary function over time, planning appropriate hormonal replacement for brain-injured patients who acquired hypopituitarism is possible. This program requires tight collaboration with rehabilitation doctors and neurosurgeons.

6. Acknowledgment

This work is supported in part by Taiwan Department of Health Clinical Trial and Research Center of Excellence (DOH100-TD-B-111-004).

7. References

(1999). "Consensus conference. Rehabilitation of persons with traumatic brain injury. NIH Consensus Development Panel on Rehabilitation of Persons With Traumatic Brain Injury." JAMA 282(10): 974-83.

Adekoya, N., D. J. Thurman, et al. (2002). "Surveillance for traumatic brain injury deaths--United States, 1989-1998." MMWR Surveill Summ 51(10): 1-14.

Agha, A., B. Rogers, et al. (2004). "Neuroendocrine dysfunction in the acute phase of traumatic brain injury." Clin Endocrinol (Oxf) 60(5): 584-91.

Agha, A., M. Sherlock, et al. (2005). "The natural history of post-traumatic neurohypophysial dysfunction." Eur J Endocrinol 152(3): 371-7.

Agha, A., E. Thornton, et al. (2004). "Posterior pituitary dysfunction after traumatic brain injury." J Clin Endocrinol Metab 89(12): 5987-92.

Aimaretti, G., M. R. Ambrosio, et al. (2004). "Traumatic brain injury and subarachnoid haemorrhage are conditions at high risk for hypopituitarism: screening study at 3 months after the brain injury." Clin Endocrinol (Oxf) 61(3): 320-6.

Bavisetty, S., D. L. McArthur, et al. (2008). "Chronic hypopituitarism after traumatic brain injury: risk assessment and relationship to outcome." Neurosurgery 62(5): 1080-93; discussion 1093-4.

Behan, L. A., J. Phillips, et al. (2008). "Neuroendocrine disorders after traumatic brain injury." J Neurol Neurosurg Psychiatry 79(7): 753-9.

Benvenga, S., A. Campenni, et al. (2000). "Clinical review 113: Hypopituitarism secondary to head trauma." J Clin Endocrinol Metab 85(4): 1353-61.

Bohn, D., M. R. Davids, et al. (2005). "Acute and fatal hyponatraemia after resection of a craniopharyngioma: a preventable tragedy." QJM 98(9): 691-703.

Bohnen, N., A. Twijnstra, et al. (1993). "Water metabolism and postconcussional symptoms 5 weeks after mild head injury." Eur Neurol 33(1): 77-9.

Bondanelli, M., L. De Marinis, et al. (2004). "Occurrence of pituitary dysfunction following traumatic brain injury." J Neurotrauma 21(6): 685-96.

Boughey, J. C., M. J. Yost, et al. (2004). "Diabetes insipidus in the head-injured patient." Am Surg 70(6): 500-3.

Brooks, B. S., T. el Gammal, et al. (1989). "Frequency and variation of the posterior pituitary bright signal on MR images." AJR Am J Roentgenol 153(5): 1033-8.

Ceballos, R. (1966). "Pituitary changes in head trauma (analysis of 102 consecutive cases of head injury)." Ala J Med Sci 3(2): 185-98.

Chou, Y. C., T. Y. Wang, et al. (2009). "Permanent central diabetes insipidus after mild traumatic brain injury." Brain Inj 23(13-14): 1095-8.

Crompton, M. R. (1971). "Hypothalamic lesions following closed head injury." Brain 94(1): 165-72.

Cytowic, R. E., A. Smith, et al. (1986). "Transient amenorrhea after closed head trauma." N Engl J Med 314(11): 715.

Dimopoulou, I., S. Tsagarakis, et al. (2004). "Endocrine abnormalities in critical care patients with moderate-to-severe head trauma: incidence, pattern and predisposing factors." Intensive Care Med 30(6): 1051-7.

Edwards, O. M. and J. D. Clark (1986). "Post-traumatic hypopituitarism. Six cases and a review of the literature." Medicine (Baltimore) 65(5): 281-90.

Estes, S. M. and R. J. Urban (2005). "Hormonal replacement in patients with brain injury-induced hypopituitarism: who, when and how to treat?" Pituitary 8(3-4): 267-70.

Ghirardello, S., N. Hopper, et al. (2006). "Diabetes insipidus in craniopharyngioma: postoperative management of water and electrolyte disorders." J Pediatr Endocrinol Metab 19 Suppl 1: 413-21.

Hadjizacharia, P., E. O. Beale, et al. (2008). "Acute diabetes insipidus in severe head injury: a prospective study." J Am Coll Surg 207(4): 477-84.

Halimi, P., R. Sigal, et al. (1988). "Post-traumatic diabetes insipidus: MR demonstration of pituitary stalk rupture." J Comput Assist Tomogr 12(1): 135-7.

Harper, C. G., D. Doyle, et al. (1986). "Analysis of abnormalities in pituitary gland in non-missile head injury: study of 100 consecutive cases." J Clin Pathol 39(7): 769-73.

Hellawell, D. J., R. T. Taylor, et al. (1999). "Cognitive and psychosocial outcome following moderate or severe traumatic brain injury." Brain Inj 13(7): 489-504.

Kelly, D. F., I. T. Gonzalo, et al. (2000). "Hypopituitarism following traumatic brain injury and aneurysmal subarachnoid hemorrhage: a preliminary report." J Neurosurg 93(5): 743-52.

Kelly, D. F., D. L. McArthur, et al. (2006). "Neurobehavioral and quality of life changes associated with growth hormone insufficiency after complicated mild, moderate, or severe traumatic brain injury." J Neurotrauma 23(6): 928-42.

Klose, M., A. Juul, et al. (2007). "Prevalence and predictive factors of post-traumatic hypopituitarism." Clin Endocrinol (Oxf) 67(2): 193-201.

Kornblum, R. N. and R. S. Fisher (1969). "Pituitary lesions in craniocerebral injuries." Arch Pathol 88(3): 242-8.

Kraus, J. F. and D. L. McArthur (1996). "Epidemiologic aspects of brain injury." Neurol Clin 14(2): 435-50.

Kuzeyli, K., E. Cakir, et al. (2001). "Diabetes insipidus secondary to penetrating spinal cord trauma: case report and literature review." Spine (Phila Pa 1976) 26(21): E510-1.

Leal-Cerro, A., J. M. Flores, et al. (2005). "Prevalence of hypopituitarism and growth hormone deficiency in adults long-term after severe traumatic brain injury." Clin Endocrinol (Oxf) 62(5): 525-32.

Levin, H. S., H. E. Gary, Jr., et al. (1990). "Neurobehavioral outcome 1 year after severe head injury. Experience of the Traumatic Coma Data Bank." J Neurosurg 73(5): 699-709.

Lieberman, S. A., A. L. Oberoi, et al. (2001). "Prevalence of neuroendocrine dysfunction in patients recovering from traumatic brain injury." J Clin Endocrinol Metab 86(6): 2752-6.

Maggiore, U., E. Picetti, et al. (2009). "The relation between the incidence of hypernatremia and mortality in patients with severe traumatic brain injury." Crit Care 13(4): R110.

Maghnie, M., G. Cosi, et al. (2000). "Central diabetes insipidus in children and young adults." N Engl J Med 343(14): 998-1007.

Maiya, B., V. Newcombe, et al. (2008). "Magnetic resonance imaging changes in the pituitary gland following acute traumatic brain injury." Intensive Care Med 34(3): 468-75.

Massol, J., P. Humbert, et al. (1987). "Post-traumatic diabetes insipidus and amenorrhea-galactorrhea syndrome after pituitary stalk rupture." Neuroradiology 29(3): 299-300.

Pierucci, G., G. Gherson, et al. (1971). "[Pituitary changes especially necrotic--following cranio-cerebral injuries]." Pathologica 63(917): 71-88.

Powner, D. J., C. Boccalandro, et al. (2006). "Endocrine failure after traumatic brain injury in adults." Neurocrit Care 5(1): 61-70.

Ray, J. G. (1998). "DDAVP use during pregnancy: an analysis of its safety for mother and child." Obstet Gynecol Surv 53(7): 450-5.

Rembratt, A., C. Graugaard-Jensen, et al. (2004). "Pharmacokinetics and pharmacodynamics of desmopressin administered orally versus intravenously at daytime versus night-time in healthy men aged 55-70 years." Eur J Clin Pharmacol 60(6): 397-402.

Rittig, S., A. R. Jensen, et al. (1998). "Effect of food intake on the pharmacokinetics and antidiuretic activity of oral desmopressin (DDAVP) in hydrated normal subjects." Clin Endocrinol (Oxf) 48(2): 235-41.

Rose, B., R. Narins, et al. (2001). "Clinical Physiology of Acid-Base and Electrolyte Disorders, 5th ed, ." 751-754.

Rouvillois, H., L. Reverchon, et al. (1921). "L´esions traumatiques del'hypophyse dans les fractures de la base du crane." Bull Mem Soc Chirurg Paris 47: 685-689.

Rutland-Brown, W., J. A. Langlois, et al. (2006). "Incidence of traumatic brain injury in the United States, 2003." J Head Trauma Rehabil 21(6): 544-8.

Salehi, F., K. Kovacs, et al. (2007). "Histologic study of the human pituitary gland in acute traumatic brain injury." Brain Inj 21(6): 651-6.

Schneider, H. J., I. Kreitschmann-Andermahr, et al. (2007). "Hypothalamopituitary dysfunction following traumatic brain injury and aneurysmal subarachnoid hemorrhage: a systematic review." JAMA 298(12): 1429-38.

Schneider, H. J., P. G. Samann, et al. (2007). "Pituitary imaging abnormalities in patients with and without hypopituitarism after traumatic brain injury." J Endocrinol Invest 30(4): RC9-RC12.

Seckl, J. and D. Dunger (1989). "Postoperative diabetes insipidus." BMJ 298(6665): 2-3.

Segal-Lieberman, G., A. Karasik, et al. (2000). "Hypopituitarism following closed head injury." Pituitary 3(3): 181-4.

Sigounas, D. G., J. L. Sharpless, et al. (2008). "Predictors and incidence of central diabetes insipidus after endoscopic pituitary surgery." Neurosurgery 62(1): 71-8; discussion 78-9.

Stenberg, A. and G. Lackgren (1994). "Desmopressin tablets in the treatment of severe nocturnal enuresis in adolescents." Pediatrics 94(6 Pt 1): 841-6.

Teasdale, G. and B. Jennett (1974). "Assessment of coma and impaired consciousness. A practical scale." Lancet 2(7872): 81-4.

Thurman, J., R. Halterman, et al. (2003). "Chapter 34. Therapy of dysnatremic disorders." Therapy in Nephrology and Hypertension, 2nd edition, Saunders, London: 335-348.

Tsagarakis, S., M. Tzanela, et al. (2005). "Diabetes insipidus, secondary hypoadrenalism and hypothyroidism after traumatic brain injury: clinical implications." Pituitary 8(3-4): 251-4.

Vokes, T. J., M. B. Gaskill, et al. (1988). "Antibodies to vasopressin in patients with diabetes insipidus. Implications for diagnosis and therapy." Ann Intern Med 108(2): 190-5.

3

Management of Neuroendocrine Instability During Maintenance of Potential Organ Donors

Luciana Mascia, Ilaria Mastromauro and Silvia Grottoli
University of Turin
Italy

1. Introduction

Solid organ transplantation is the treatment of choice for patients with end-stage cardiac, pulmonary or liver disease. This form of surgical treatment has enjoyed increasing success, with better early and late survival for lung, liver and cardiac transplantation, while renal transplantation is both cost effective and improves the quality of life for the recipient receiving dialysis. The main limiting factor for this successful procedure is the shortage of suitable donor organs, resulting in longer waiting list for patients with a substantial risk of mortality before transplantation (Keegan M.T. 2009).

The majority of organs come from patients who suffered an acute neurologic injury, such as traumatic brain injury or cerebrovascular accidents, including spontaneous intracerebral bleeding and thrombosis that progresses to brainstem death. Unfortunately, not all brainstem dead patients become potential organ donors and organ are ultimately harvested from only 15-20% of individuals who satisfy organ donor criteria (Mascia et al 2010). Many reasons contribute to the paucity of donor organs, such as the sub-optimal critical care management of potential organ donors, lack of consent, logistical problems and the use of strict donor criteria (Mascia et al 2006).

In the present chapter we will discuss neuroendocrine alterations which occur in acute brain injured patients evolving to brain death. Since most of the data available has been collected in acute neurological patients with varying impairment of the conscious state, we will first summarize the pathophysiology, clinical signs, diagnosis and treatment of endocrine abnormalities in severe brain injury patients and then we will focus on the consequences of neuroendocrine alterations in brain dead subjects. These abnormalities contribute to the hemodynamic and metabolic instability of the potential organ donors and may affect organs availability for transplantation.

In severe acute brain injury patients evolving to brain death, hypothalamic-pituitary-adrenal insufficiency occurs in 30-50% (Behan et al 2008; Corneli et al 2007) of patients and a high prevalence of neuroendocrine deficiency is present in brain dead patients (Howlett et al 1989; Salim et al 2006). These endocrine alterations lead to metabolic abnormalities and hemodynamic instability with deleterious effects on these potential organ donors (Ullah et al 2006). Adequate organ donor management is therefore mandatory to prevent, reduce or reverse these alterations and to maintain the functional integrity of potentially transplantable organs. Since all donors are treated in intensive care units an optimal clinical management would be an integral component of intensive care medicine education and practice. Nevertheless a substantial variability between medical centres and a consequent sub-optimal clinical management exists in the field of organ donors treatment (Mascia et al 2009). Regarding the neuroendocrine alterations most of the studies have been performed in neurological patients looking at the long term effects of these abnormalities.

When we treat acute neurological patients with a preserved conscious status who develop endocrine alterations such as anti-diuretic hormone depletion, details from the clinical history are collected, symptoms developed over time frame of weeks or even months are recorded, then clinical signs are identified and laboratory tests are required to confirm the clinical diagnosis. Finally a therapeutic strategy is implemented and the clinical prognosis is proposed according to the severity of symptoms and signs as well as the response to treatment. When we treat acute neurological patients with a severe impairment in the conscious state and endocrine alterations, the clinical history, symptoms and signs are not easily evaluated, although severe hemodynamic and metabolic alterations usually occur in a time frame of hours or few days. Laboratory tests are required to confirm the clinical diagnosis, a therapeutic strategies must be readily implemented and the severity of clinical status will have a prognostic value. When we treat potential organ donors with neuroendocrine alterations, clinical signs develop within minutes or few hours with a dramatic impairment in systemic hemodynamics and metabolism. Therefore, clinical diagnosis, laboratory test confirmation and implementation of the specific therapy are required in a time frame of minutes or few hours. Moreover, no prognostic evaluation is required, while hemodynamic stability and prompt correction of metabolic alterations are mandatory in order to guarantee an optimal organ perfusion and metabolic homeostasis for organ donation.

2. Neuroendocrine alterations in severe acute neurological patients

Several studies have demonstrated that brain injury such as traumatic brain injury (TBI) or subarachnoid hemorrhage (SAH) is a frequent cause of hypopituitarism, with an incidence that is much greater than previously reported.

First of all, we have to introduce a distinction between acute and prolonged critical illness in term of metabolic and neuroendocrine paradigms. The initial endocrine response consists primarily of an activated release of anterior pituitary hormone and peripheral inactivation of anabolic pathways. In the chronic phase there is a uniformly impaired pulsatile secretion of anterior pituitary hormones at least in part due to hypothalamic origin (Van den Berghe et al 1998), which is correlated with reduced activity of target tissue. However, this specific pituitary-dependent axis can be reactivated with preserved peripheral responsiveness. Another mandatory issue to underline is that there is sufficient data from the literature concerning long term effects at hypothalamic or pituitary level of TBI or SAH, while data regarding the short term effects of severe acute neurological injuries in terms of neuroendocrine activity are very scanty.

The first report of TBI-induced hypopituitarism was published in 1918 (Cyran 1918). Then several retrospective studies and case reports identified additional conditions of hypopituitarism following head injury (Altman and Pruzanski 1961; Edwards and Clark 1986; Kusanagi et al 2000). In particular, more than ten years ago Benvenga et al. confirmed the relationship between TBI and hypopituitarism (Benvenga et al 2000). These authors reported that in 70% of cases hypopituitarism was diagnosed within 1 year of injury. Indeed there are reports of patients with total, multiple or isolated hypopituitarism whose clinical history revealed the occurrence of TBI many years before the diagnosis.

Subarachnoid hemorrhage produces a pattern of deficits similar to that of TBI. Patients with aneurysmal SAH frequently present persistent physical, psychosocial, cognitive and emotional deficits similar to those of patients with untreated partial or complete hypopituitarism, even if clinicians do not normally relate these symptoms to pituitary insufficiency.

In the field of intensive care medicine, several studies show that critically ill patients with TBI frequently exhibited an abnormal pituitary hormonal response in the immediate post-injury period (Agha et al 2004b; Aimaretti et al 2004; Bondanelli et al 2005; Dimopoulou et al 2004). On the other hand, the critical illness itself has profound effects on the pituitary function (Van den Berghe and de Zegher 1996) that is characterized by protein hypercatabolism, preservations of fat depots and immune dysfunction. Since the anterior pituitary gland is the first regulator of human metabolism and immune function, the presence of an extensive interaction between these three players is not surprising. Interestingly, the critical illness may be associated with reduced levels of activity in the different pituitary axes, except for the corticotropic axis (Van den Berghe and de Zegher 1996). Furthermore, in the critical care scenario some therapeutic strategies such as the infusion of dopamine has been found to be associated with an impaired pituitary function, which has raised the hypothesis that dopamine may play a role in the pathogenesis of the pituitary dysfunction present in critical illness (Van den Berghe and de Zegher 1996).

2.1 Epidemiology

TBI-related hypopituitarism remains largely under-diagnosed, mostly due to the lack of awareness among physicians who take care of these patients. Indeed, considering the epidemiology of TBI (91–332/100,000 inhabitants all over the world) and the high risk to develop the most severe form of multiple or total hypopituitarism (at least 10–15% of patients), it has became more evident that many patients misdiagnosed hypopituitarism induced by brain injury may experience a poor quality of life and a low life expectancy.

The estimated incidence rates for SAH are between 10 to 25 per 100,000 per year. Morbidity and mortality in the acute phase are due to the pathophysiological changes related to the initial bleeding, such as the abrupt increase in intracranial pressure, impairment of cerebral perfusion and focal or global cerebral ischemia. In studies which included both SAH and TBI patients, an incidence different degrees of hypopituitarism was reported to be 27% and 47% respectively (Schneider et al 2007).

2.2 Pathophysiology

Pituitary function is at particular risk because of the vulnerable anatomic location of the gland within the sella turcica as well as its delicate infundibular hypothalamic structure and its fragile vascular supply (Kelly et al 2000). In several neuropathological studies haemorrhage, necrosis, and fibrosis of the pituitary gland and hypothalamus have been recorded after TBI or SAH. Stalk lesions can produce anterior-lobe infarction by damaging the portal blood supply (Daniel et al 1959; Kornblum and Fisher 1969). Hypothalamic lesions consisting of areas of ischemic necrosis, macro and micro-haemorrhages were noted in two-thirds of the patients who died shortly after SAH (Bondanelli et al 2006).

Growth hormonal deficiency is most often seen in patients with TBI since the growth hormone-secreting somatotrope cells are located in the wings of the pituitary gland and the vascular supply and oxygen they receive come out of the hypothalamic-pituitary portal vessels. Consequently, damage in this area impairs the blood and oxygen supply, resulting in cell death. In contrast, the cells that secrete adrenocorticotropin hormone and thyroid-stimulating hormone are located ventrally in the more protected, medial portion of the pituitary, and they receive blood from the portal vessels and the anterior pituitary artery branch, which provides nutrients and oxygen to this area and to all the cells located in the sub-capsular part (Kelly et al 2000). However, data from literature show that the frequency of growth hormone deficiency and low cortisol levels are 15% and 46% respectively in TBI while in SAH the risk of hypopituitarism may be even higher (Agha et al 2004b; Aimaretti et al 2004; Casanueva et al 2004; Kreitschmann-Andermahr et al 2004).

Disorders of salt and water balance, in particular diabetes insipidus (DI) and the syndrome of inappropriate antidiuretic hormone secretion, are common complications in the acute phase of TBI (Kaufman et al 1993). Available information on the frequency of post-traumatic DI are mainly derived from retrospective data (Boughey et al 2004; Wong et al 1998), while few prospective studies have accurately defined the natural history of DI following TBI. In the first prospective study Agha and collegues (Agha et al 2005) investigated the sequential posterior pituitary function after TBI and reported a frequency of early post-traumatic DI equal to 26%. Further studies reported a negative correlation between Glasgow Coma Scale and plasmatic levels of both osmolality and sodium, and a positive correlation between Glasgow Coma Scale and peak urine osmolality in the acute phase of TBI, suggesting that acute DI is associated with the severity of injury. Post-traumatic DI may result from inflammatory oedema around the hypothalamus or posterior pituitary, with recovery as the swelling resolves. It can also result from direct damage to the paraventricular and supraoptic hypothalamic neurones, the pituitary stalk or axon terminals in the posterior pituitary. These abnormalities may be either transient, if the supraoptic and paraventricular neurones form new vascular connections, or become permanent if gliosis occurs (Yuan and Wade 1991).

Finally, pituitary function is impaired in 50% of patients with primary brain tumors, as a consequence of surgery and radiotherapy. Hypopituitarism in patients with primary brain tumors often includes severe growth hormone deficiency. However, the efficacy of treatment of hypopituitarism in patients with primary brain tumours has never been demonstrated (Schneider et al 2006).

2.3 Clinical signs and symptoms of hypopituitarism

In acute neurological patients with a preserved conscious level hypopituitarism is associated with a number of non-specific signs and symptoms. Fatigue is a major symptom (Kreutzer et al 2001; LaChapelle and Finlayson 1998) although this symptom may also be related to TBI. Other signs, symptoms and laboratory abnormalities include decreased lean body mass with increased body fat and dyslipidaemia, reduced exercise tolerance and muscle strength (Carroll et al 1998), DI (Edwards and Clark 1986), decreased thyroid-stimulating hormone and free tyroxine levels and adrenal insufficiency (Benvenga et al 2000; Carroll et al 1998; Lieberman et al 2001), amenorrhea/infertility, erectile dysfunction and hyperprolactinaemia (Benvenga et al 2000; Cytowic et al 1986), diminished cardiovascular function, impaired cognitive function, memory loss, decreased concentration, mood disturbances, increased anxiety and depression, irritability, insomnia (Deijen et al 1996; Howlett et al 1989; Leon-Carrion et al 2001) and a feeling of social isolation (Carroll et al 1998). A deficiency of growth hormone produces metabolic effects in different organs with consequences in both physical and emotional areas. These signs and symptoms of hypopituitarism are the same in hypopituitaric patients after TBI. These symptoms and signs of hypopituitarism are also present in TBI in the sub-acute phase. The overlap of clinical manifestations due to the sequelae of TBI or to the presence of hypopituitarism induced by trauma may result in a sub-optimal rehabilitation of TBI patients with hypopituitarism.

Traditionally, the onset of DI was considered a useful indicator of hypopituitarism because it is routinely attributed to pituitary insult. However, reports of the incidence of DI following brain injury vary widely, with Benvenga et al. (Benvenga et al 2000) reporting as many as 30% of cases compared to Aimaretti et al. (Aimaretti et al 2004) who reported only 5.5%. In a recent retrospective study, the incidence of severe hypernatremic cases of DI was 2.9% but the incidence of less severe forms seems to be much higher. Agha et al, in a retrospective study reported an incidence of 21.6% in the immediate period following TBI, which was related to the severity of the traumatic insult but not related to the development of anterior pituitary abnormalities (Agha et al 2004a). The discrepancy between anterior and posterior pituitary altered function has been recently confirmed in a prospective study which reported a high incidence of DI (26%) (Agha et al 2004a).

Likewise, reports on the incidence of hyperprolactinaemia, another marker of hypothalamus-pituitary derangement, following brain injury vary even more dramatically (Aimaretti et al 2004; Benvenga et al 2000; Lieberman et al 2001). While these findings provide evidence that TBI is associated with derangement of the hypothalamus-pituitary unit, it underscores the fact that a full endocrinologic assessment is necessary to determine the extent of the hormonal alterations after TBI and the need for a global endocrine evaluation. Aimaretti and co-workers (Aimaretti et al 2005) in a multicentered study prospectively investigated the risk to develop hypopituitarism in brain injured patients. Pituitary function was evaluated in 100 patients with TBI and in 40 patients with SAH after 3 and 12 months to evaluate the incidence of hypopituitarism and the effect of pituitary deficits on outcome one year after the brain injury. The 3 month study showed some degree of hypopituitarism in 35% of TBI patients. Total, multiple and isolated deficits were present in 4, 6 and 25% respectively. DI was present in 4%, secondary adrenal, thyroid and gonadal deficit was present in 8, 5 and 17%, respectively. Severe growth hormone deficiency was the most frequent pituitary defect (25%). In SAH patients some degree of hypopituitarism was reported in 37.5%. Multiple and isolated deficits were present in 10 and 27.5% respectively. DI was present in 7.5%, secondary adrenal, thyroid and gonadal deficits was present in 2.5, 7.5 and 12.5%, respectively. Severe growth hormone deficiency was the most frequent defect (25%). The 12 months retesting demonstrated that some degree of hypopituitarism was still present in 22.7% of the TBI patients. Total hypopituitarism was always confirmed at 12 months while multiple and isolated hypopituitarism was confirmed in 25%, DI was present in 2.8%. In SAH after 12 months retesting hypopituitarism was present in 37.5% with multiple or isolated deficits in 6.2 and 31.3% respectively. No multiple deficits were confirmed at 12 months but in 2 patients new deficits were diagnosed. It is important to note that 30.7% of SAH with isolated deficits at 3 months displayed normal pituitary function at 12 months and the most common deficit was severe growth hormone deficiency in both TBI and SAH.

These data indicate that pituitary function may improve over time and that hypopituitarism is transient in most cases and would reflect effective repair of the hypothalamic-pituitary damage induced by brain injuries.

Considering the topic of this chapter it is important to note that the acute phase is characterized by a high incidence of hypopituitarism as sign of the acute brain damage in the hypothalamic pituitary area.

2.4 Diagnosis

Diagnosis of hypopituitarism due to brain injury does not differ from that of hypopituitarism due to other causes. Test of pituitary hormones function and their target glands should be always performed.

Diabetes insipidus is demonstrated by the presence of massive dilute urine volume (>3 L/24 h) with low urine osmolality (<300 mmol/kg) (Aimaretti et al 1998a; Aimaretti et al 1998b; Lamberts et al 1998; Lissett CA 1996).

Secondary adrenal insufficiency is demonstrated by early-morning (at 9:00 am) cortisol concentrations less than 30 μg/L (or < 100 pmol/L) and morning ACTH below upper reference range, associated with another pituitary deficit (Aimaretti et al 1998a; Aimaretti et al 1998b; Lamberts et al 1998; Lissett CA 1996).

Secondary hypothyroidism is demonstrated by low free tyroxine (<8 ng/l) concentrations with normal or low thyroid-stimulating hormone levels (Aimaretti et al 1998a; Aimaretti et al 1998b; Lamberts et al 1998; Lissett CA 1996).

Secondary hypogonadism is demonstrated by: (1) in premenopausal women low estradiol levels (<20 pg/ml) with normal or low follicle-stimulating hormone and luteinizing hormone levels; (2) in men by low testosterone levels (<3 µg/l) with low or normal follicle-stimulating hormone and luteinizing hormone levels (Aimaretti et al 1998a; Aimaretti et al 1998b; Lamberts et al 1998; Lissett CA 1996).

GH deficiency is demonstrated by peak growth hormone response to growth hormone releasing hormone + arginine below 16.5 µg/L (3rd centile limit of normal growth hormone response). A peak growth hormone response below 9.0 µg/L (1st centile limit) indicates severe growth hormone deficiency (Aimaretti et al 1998a; Ghigo et al 2001; Lamberts et al 1998). Insulin-like growth factor-I levels were considered with respect to the 25th centile age-related normal limits (Aimaretti et al 1998a; Ghigo et al 2001; Hartman et al 2002; Lamberts et al 1998). From an endocrinological point of view, TBI patients in coma or in vegetative state should not be evaluated. The reason is that no data are now available showing that an early diagnosis and appropriate replacement for the different forms of hypopituitarism can be of any benefit for patients in such extreme conditions.

Therefore endocrinologists should perform a neuroendocrine assessment in: 1) patients who develop an acute form of hypopituitarism in the early phases after TBI (i.e. DI and electrolyte abnormalities in particular) 2) patients with abnormalities in the brain imaging techniques like hemorrhagic lesions (on CT or MRI scan). Although a neuroendocrine assessment is not a priority in severe neurological patients, an optimal hemodynamic management of severe brain injured patients is crucial to guarantee adequate perfusion to the brain during the repair process. Therefore, a prompt diagnosis and treatment of anti-diuretic hormone, cortisol and insulin depletion in severe brain injured patients may play a relevant role in stabilizing hemodynamic and electrolyte abnormalities. When these patients evolve to brain death hemodynamic stability remains a crucial part of the clinical management to optimize peripheral organ perfusion.

2.5 Therapeutic strategy

2.5.1 Who

The severity of TBI or SAH has been suggested as a risk factor for the development of hypopituitarism. Although some discrepancies are present in the literature, the degree of severity of the brain lesion is considered a limiting factor for treatment of endocrine abnormalities. Kelly et al. (Kelly et al 2000) identified Glasgow coma scale scores < 10, diffuse brain swelling on initial CT and hypotensive or hypoxic insults as significant predictors for the development of hypopituitarism. Bondanelli et al. (Bondanelli et al 2004) confirmed that hypopituitarism was more prevalent in TBI patients with low Glasgow coma scale although the CT scan abnormalities based on the Marshall classification did not predict the development of pituitary abnormalities. Indeed, Lieberman et al (Lieberman et al 2001) and Aimaretti et al. (Aimaretti et al 2004; Aimaretti et al 2005) did not confirm any correlation between Glasgow coma scale and pituitary dysfunction. Because of these discrepancies regarding the risk factors for pituitary abnormalities after TBI, it is difficult to identify which patients should be screened for these alterations. However it is well known that: 1) hemodynamic instability (hypotension and low cerebral perfusion) and electrolyte abnormalities may affect neurological outcome after TBI; and 2) pituitary abnormalities may have a relevant impact on hemodynamic and metabolic homeostasis. Therefore, in order to guarantee the optimal clinical management of severe brain injured patients it is wise to plan a basic screening test for the presence of endocrine abnormalities after TBI.

2.5.2 When

It is well known that hormonal secretion from the pituitary is altered immediately following TBI (Chiolero and Berger 1994). However, because of the use of drugs, metabolic abnormalities, and functional alterations, a condition of hypopituitarism is difficult to assess (Dimopoulou et al 2004). Agha et al. (Agha et al 2004a) examined the prevalence of anterior and posterior pituitary dysfunction in the acute (7–21 days) phase following TBI. The authors identified adrenocorticotropin hormone deficiency and posterior pituitary dysfunction as the main abnormalities which required immediate replacement therapy. In the recovery phase, Aimaretti et al. (Aimaretti et al 2004; Aimaretti et al 2005) established that early diagnosis of pan-hypopituitarism is always confirmed at one year and thus treatment is required at the time of diagnosis. In the chronic phase, Bondanelli et al. (Bondanelli et al 2004) observed a high prevalence of growth hormonal deficiency and hypogonadotrophic hypogonadism but not corticotrophic and posterior dysfunction.

2.5.3 How

To date there are no conclusive data on this topic in severe brain injured patients. In cases with a clear indication of hormonal deficiency, the treatment should be conducted by an endocrinologist as defined by the international guidelines. DI, adrenal insufficiency, thyroid dysfunction and hypogonadism should be treated along with appropriate follow up.

Diabetes insipidus The general goals of treatment are the correction of pre-existing water deficits and reduction in ongoing excessive urinary water losses; however, the specific therapy varies with the clinical situation. Ambulatory patients with DI and normal thirst have little body water deficit and may be helped from relief of the polyuria and polydipsia that disrupt normal activities. In contrast, comatose patients with or without DI are unable to drink in response to thirst, and in these patients progressive hypertonicity may be a life-threatening situation. A variety of anti-diuretic agents have been used to treat central DI, but desmopressina is the treatment of choice for this disorder. Desmopressina is an anti-diuretic hormone analogue, which particularly useful because it has a much longer half-life than anti-diuretic hormone and is devoid of the pressor activity of anti-diuretic hormone at vascular V1 receptors. Desmopressina is generally administered orally (60-120 μg every 8–

24 hours), but can be given parenterally in acute situations (1–2 mg intravenously, intramuscularly or subcutaneously). For both oral and parenteral preparations, the increase of the administered dose generally has the effect to prolong the duration of anti-diuresis rather than increasing its magnitude; consequently, altering the dose can be useful to reduce the required frequency of administration. Synthetic anti-diuretic hormone (Pitressin) can also be used to treat central DI, but its use is limited by a much shorter half-life, requiring frequent doses or a continuous infusion, and carries a side effect of increased blood pressure due to vasoconstriction.

Secondary adrenal insufficiency Conventional treatment is represented by 10–25 mg of hydrocortisone per day (2–3 doses per day) or 25–37.5 mg of cortisone acetate. It is essential to use the lowest possible dose. In stress situations (psyco-emotional, surgery, transient diseases, infections etc.) the dose should be increased to 25-50 hydrocortisone per day or 50-75 mg of cortisone acetate or if reduction of intestinal absorption is expected parenteral hydrocortisone 100-50 mg should be administered.

Secondary hypothyroidism L-thyroxine is considered the drug of choice. The usual replacement dose is age-dependent and varies from 1.3 μg/kg (< 60 yrs) to 1.1 μg/kg (> 60 yrs). The most common route of administration is oral, even through nasogastric tube, but in acute situations when this is not possible, parenteral administration can be used (50-300 μg/daily iv). Because thyroid hormone replacement increases the rate of metabolism of glucocorticoids, which can lead to an adrenal crisis, replacement therapy should begin after hydrocortisone substitution has been initiated.

Hypogonadism In male patients testosterone substitution (testosterone gel 25–50 mg/day or testosterone undecanoate 1000 mg every 3 months) returned bone and muscle mass, sexual function and haematocrit to normal levels.

In pre-menopausal female patients sex hormone substitution (20–35 μg ethinyl oestradiol or oestradiol valerate 2–4 mg/day plus progesterone unless hysterectomised) can return libido, well being and bone mass to normal levels. In post menopausal women sex hormone therapy is not indicated because a significant increased risk of cardiovascular and neoplastic diseases.

3. Neuroendocrine alterations in brain dead patients

Brain death results from damage to the brain stem with a complete irreversible loss of its function. This devastating insult to the brain stem is immediately followed by a "sympathetic storm". In addition, brain death causes significant endocrine alterations involving the hypothalamic-pituitary axis and triggers an inflammatory reaction. The catecholamine storm, the endocrine disturbances and the systemic inflammatory reaction represent the first insult with consequential organ insufficiency and metabolic derangement (Avlonitis et al 2003). Sub-optimal management of potential organ donors leading to a further impairment of the cardiovascular and respiratory function represents an additional damage to potentially transplantable organs (Fisher et al 1999; Venkateswaran et al 2009a). Any intervention in each of these three phases in order to prevent or treat these insults may have an impact on the functional outcome of transplanted organs (figure 1). In this prospective a prompt recognition and treatment of neuroendocrine alterations represent one of the possible therapeutic strategies able to optimise organ availability for transplantation.

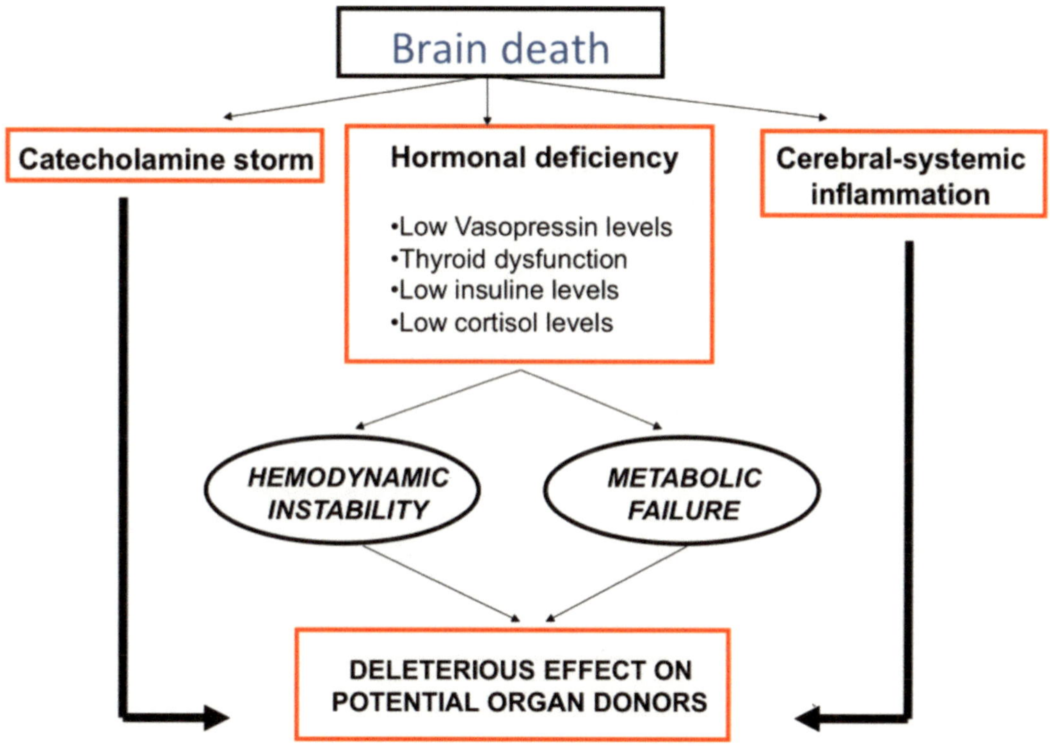

Fig. 1. Pathophysiology of hormonal deficiency in brain death and its implication on organ donors maintainance

3.1 Pathophysiology

Brain death has an important impact on endocrine function leading to profound metabolic abnormalities and hemodynamic instability with deleterious effects on the potential organ donors (Chamorro et al 2009; Smith 2004). The most important endocrine disturbances are a reduction in anti-diuretic hormone secretion, thyroid dysfunction, reduction in adenocorticotrophic hormone and insulin levels (Ullah et al 2006). In experimental animal models of brain death, the pituitary gland hormones vasopressin and adenocorticotrophic hormone decreased significantly after 15 and 45 minutes of brain death respectively (Bittner et al 1995). Circulating triiodothyronine, thyroxine, glucagons and insulin concentrations were significantly reduced within a few hours after brain death (Bittner et al 1995; Chen et al 1996). The significant reduction in circulating concentrations of stress hormones was associated with a severe hemodynamic instability (Chen et al 1996; Hing et al 2007; Novitzky et al 2006). In a prospective randomized experimental study of brain death, Hing et al. showed that hormonal replacement therapy including triiodothyronine, methylprednisolone, vasopressin and insulin reduced norepinephrine requirements and improved hemodynamics and cardiac function (Hing et al 2007).

An interesting study by Ishikawa et al. (Ishikawa et al 2009) compared, in autoptic cases, morphological results as well as endocrine function in brain death (within 24 hours post mortem), acute death (< 3 h) and delayed death (survival time 4-51 days). Histology and electronic microscopy of pituitary gland were performed and blood as well as cerebrospinal fluid levels of adrenocorticotropin hormone, growth hormone and thyroid-stimulating hormone were measured. Morphological and microscopic studies revealed partial necrosis of central anterior lobe but preservation of its periphery, autolysis in the hypothalamus, swelling of mitochondria and dilation of smooth endoplasmatic reticulum and golgi apparatus suggesting that pituitary is preserved without blood supply after brain death but the integrity of hypothalamus pituitary axis is lost. Regarding pituitary secretion, no peculiar findings were demonstrated after brain death different from cases of delayed death. In fact, serum adrenocorticotropin hormone levels were similar to the clinical reference values in both brain death, acute or delayed death cases, while serum growth hormone, cerebralspinal fluid growth hormone and adrenocorticotropin hormone levels were lower in brain and delayed death than in acute cases and serum thyroid-stimulating hormone levels were comparable in both brain death and delayed death cases (Ishikawa et al 2009).

In observational clinical studies, an early depletion of arginine vasopressin and development of DI is present in almost 45-80% of brain death organ donors (Gramm et al 1992; Howlett et al 1989; Salim et al 2006). Arginine vasopressin is one of the most important endogenously released stress hormones. It is also named anti-diuretic hormone based on its effects on the distal tubule of the kidney. It is synthesized in the hypothalamus and released into the bloodstream from posterior pituitary. Vasopressin has several important physiological functions including water retention by the V2 receptors on the kidney and constriction by V1 receptors on vascular smooth muscle on the systemic and pulmonary circulation. In addition to its anti-diuretic action, vasopressin is important in maintaining arterial blood pressure during episodes of hypotension (Gordon et al 2010). In brain dead patients there is a deficiency of vasopressin levels in systemic circulation due to supraventricular and paraventricular hypothalamic nuclei ischaemia (Agha et al 2007) or pituitary stalk damage that disrupts the hypothalamic pituitary axis associated to a defect in the baroreflex-mediated secretion of vasopressin levels in systemic circulation (Chen et al 1999; Gordon et al 2010). Therefore, the depletion of vasopressin may contribute to the hemodynamic instability associated with diabetes insipidus. In brain dead patients, low dose arginine vasopressin infusion, in addition to treating diabetes insipidus, results in significant reduction of inotropic support and has been associated with good kidney, liver and heart graft function (Pennefather et al 1995). Comparing the treatment of brain-dead patients with epinephrine alone versus epinephrine plus vasopressin the authors obtained a prolonged hemodynamic stabilization in brain-dead donors treated with vasopressin (Yoshioka et al 1986). In brain dead patients without clinical signs of DI, Chen et al obtained a significant reduction in cathecolamine doses (dopamine and/or norepinephrine) using arginine vasopressin at low dosage (0.04 to 1.0 U/min) with a significant increase in mean arterial pressure and better organ perfusion (Chen et al 1999). A complete weaning from catecholamine has been demonstrated in up to 40% of the donors with the use of vasopressin. Indeed a more extensive use of vasopressin as an alternative to norepinephrine has been suggested in a prospective randomised double blind trial (Venkateswaran et al 2009b).

Thyroid dysfunction is another event of brain death. This decrease of thyroid function is not caused by a primary failure of the thyroid or pituitary glands. It has been defined "sick euthyroid syndrome" and has also been described in cardiopulmonary by-pass. It is postulated that proinflammatory cytokines may play a role in inhibiting the conversion of thyroxine to the active form of thyroid hormone, and instead, convert it to the non-active form, reverse- thyroid hormone (Ullah et al 2006). In an animal model of brain death, Novitzky et al. showed that levels of thyroid hormones were severely depleted (Novitzky et al 1988). In interventional clinical studies the following results have been reported: 1) administration of thyroid hormone to donor and recipient improved cardiac allograph function; 2) therapy with thyroid hormone reversed donor myocardial dysfunction, promoted hemodynamic stability and reduced inotropic support (Novitzky et al 1990; Salim et al 2001). However a randomized clinical trial in a small number of potential organ donors using low dose of thyroid hormone was unable to confirm the positive effect of hormonal therapy on cardiac function (Goarin et al 1996). Conversely, in pediatric patients following cardiac surgery triidothyronine administration improved cardiac function (Bettendorf et al 2000). Therefore, there is still a considerable debate whether the sick euthyroid syndrome requires treatment.

Insulin levels fall after brain stem death, leading to a decrease in intracellular glucose concentration, the development of an cellular energy deficit, and a shift toward anaerobic metabolism and acidosis (Ullah et al 2006).

In brain dead patients there is also a significant decreases in cortisol levels that, in association with decreases in thyroid hormone, may contribute to the cardiovascular instability. The decrease in plasma cortisol may be associated with a decrease in the release of its stimulating factors adrenocorticotropic hormone from the anterior lobe of the pituitary gland (Gramm et al 1992). High dose steroid administration has a beneficial role in attenuating the effects of pro-inflammatory cytokines released after brain death. Steroids significantly improved oxygenation and simultaneously increased lung recovery (Follette et al 1998). A beneficial effect is described also in cases of liver transplantation involving donor treatment with methylprednisolone (Kotsch et al 2008).

3.2 Therapy of neuroendocrine dysfunction in potential organ donors

Several studies have suggested that the use of Hormonal Replacement Therapy (HRT) in donor management may serve a crucial role in helping to maintain metabolic stability and prevent hemodynamic instability (Rosendale et al 2003b). Rosendale et al. showed an increase of the mean number of organs from HRT donors (22.5%) when compared to non-hormonal resuscitation donors, which led to a significant increase in organs transplanted per donor (Rosendale et al 2003a; Rosendale et al 2003b). HRT allowed substantial improvement in mean arterial pressure and consequently in organ prefusion, and left ventricular stroke work index combined with reduction in central venous and wedge pressure and a reduction of inotropic support (Wheeldon et al 1995).

The selection of donors who are predicted to benefit from HRT was outlined at the Cristal City Consensus Conference Report (Rosengard et al 2002). After conventional management to adjust volume status, anemia and metabolic abnormalities, the guidelines recommended to perform an echocardiogram to rule out the structural abnormalities and document the ejection fraction. If the ejection fraction is less than 45%, a pulmonary artery catheter should be placed and HRT should be started. The four hormones commonly used are: methylprednisolone, triiodothyronine, arginine vasopressin titrated to obtain systemic vascular resistances of 800-1200 dynes/sec-cm) and insulin titrated to maintain blood sugar at 120 to 180 mg/dL (Rosengard et al 2002). However the use of HRT is not supported by a strong level of evidence. Clinical studies of HRT have been observational, retrospective, used non-matched controls and tested single hormonal replacement or a combination of

HRT but not the complete hormonal replacement advocated in the United Network for Organ Sharing guidelines (http://www.ccdt:ca/english/home.html ; Rosendale et al 2003a; Rosendale et al 2003b; Rostron et al 2008; Venkateswaran et al 2009a; Venkateswaran et al 2009b). In addition, the contribution of other changes in donor management such as invasive hemodynamic monitoring make it difficult to judge the relative contribution of combined hormonal resuscitation to the improvements in donor organs outcome reported in these studies. These observations have provided the foundation for prospective clinical trials to examine the efficacy and optimal timing of HRT. However, until these results are not available it remains prudent to reserve HRT for unstable donors requiring high doses of dopamine or with an ejection fraction of less than 45% (Rosengard et al 2002; Wood et al 2004; Zaroff et al 2002).

The diagnosis of DI in brain death patients does not differ from other clinical situations. DI must be differentiated from the polyuria induced by mannitol, hyperglicemia or diuretic agents. Assessment of diuresis (> 40 ml/kg body weight/day or 3000 cc/day), plasma (> 295 mOsm/kg) and urine (< 200 Osm/kg) osmolality and sodium levels (> 146 mEq/l) are key elements for its diagnosis (Mascia et al 2009). Plasma anti-diuretic hormone levels have little importance due to the poor reliability of the assay, the extreme high variability of anti-diuretic hormone plasma levels and the relatively long turn-around time (4–10 days) for results. The clinical goals are primarily based on the stabilization of the volume status by hypotonic fluid replacement with 5% dextrose or nasogastric water, serum sodium and osmolality and then on an adequate urine output. When urine volume loss are large, anti-diuretic hormone replacement therapy is required (Mascia et al 2009). A vasopressin infusion acts on the V1 and V2 receptors and induces vasoconstriction and anti-diuretic effects (Mutlu and Factor 2004). Low dose arginine vasopressin decreases serum osmolarity and sodium levels, maintains blood pressure and reduces the need for vasoactive medications in potential organ donors, with no deleterious short-term or long-term effects on the function of the donated kidney to the recipient (Guesde et al 1998; Rosendale et al 2003a; Wood et al 2004). Intermittent treatment with synthetic analogue anti-diuretic hormone desmopressin can also be used. Synthetic analogue anti-diuretic hormone desmopressin was synthesized as a selective antagonist of vasopressin V2 receptors. In brain death patients synthetic analogue anti-diuretic hormone desmopressin is administered parenterally (1–2 mg intravenously, intramuscularly or subcutaneously); increasing the administered dose generally has the effect of prolonging the duration of anti-diuresis rather than increasing its magnitude (Wood et al 2004).

4. Conclusion

In conclusion, hypothalamic-pituitary-adrenal insufficiency occurs in 30-50% of patients after traumatic and non-traumatic brain injury and has a high prevalence in brain dead patients. These endocrine alterations lead to metabolic abnormalities and hemodynamic instability with deleterious effects on potential organ donors. To optimize clinical management of potential organ donors and therefore guarantee the availability of transplantable organs, recent guidelines advocate the use of standardized hormonal therapy (l-thyroxine, methylprednisolone, vasopressin and insulin). This replacement therapy is suggested to stabilize brain death patients who present hemodynamic instability unresponsive to standard cardiovascular treatment. Despite available experimental data and increased interest for HRT in the management of potential organ donors, there are no prospective randomized controlled clinical studies testing combined HRT and examining its effects on donor cardiac function, hemodynamics and vasopressor requirements. Therefore in our opinion the HRT with particular attention to the antidiuretic hormone represents a valid component of the treatment choices to stabilize hemodynamics in potential organ donors. In the sub-group of brain death patients with a clear diagnosis of DI, the replacement therapy with low dose of arginine vasopressin is the treatment of choice.

5. References

Agha A, Rogers B, Mylotte D, Taleb F, Tormey W, Phillips J, Thompson CJ (2004a) Neuroendocrine dysfunction in the acute phase of traumatic brain injury. *Clin Endocrinol (Oxf)* 60:584-91

Agha A, Thornton E, O'Kelly P, Tormey W, Phillips J, Thompson CJ (2004b) Posterior pituitary dysfunction after traumatic brain injury. *J Clin Endocrinol Metab* 89:5987-92

Agha A, Sherlock M, Phillips J, Tormey W, Thompson CJ (2005) The natural history of post-traumatic neurohypophysial dysfunction. *Eur J Endocrinol* 152:371-7

Agha A, Phillips J, Thompson CJ (2007) Hypopituitarism following traumatic brain injury (TBI). *Br J Neurosurg* 21:210-6

Aimaretti G, Corneli G, Razzore P, Bellone S, Baffoni C, Arvat E, Camanni F, Ghigo E (1998a) Comparison between insulin-induced hypoglycemia and growth hormone (GH)-releasing hormone + arginine as provocative tests for the diagnosis of GH deficiency in adults. *J Clin Endocrinol Metab* 83:1615-8

Aimaretti G, Corneli G, Razzore P, Bellone S, Baffoni C, Bellone J, Camanni F, Ghigo E (1998b) Usefulness of IGF-I assay for the diagnosis of GH deficiency in adults. *J Endocrinol Invest* 21:506-11

Aimaretti G, Ambrosio MR, Di Somma C, Fusco A, Cannavo S, Gasperi M, Scaroni C, De Marinis L, Benvenga S, degli Uberti EC, Lombardi G, Mantero F, Martino E, Giordano G, Ghigo E (2004) Traumatic brain injury and subarachnoid haemorrhage are conditions at high risk for hypopituitarism: screening study at 3 months after the brain injury. *Clin Endocrinol (Oxf)* 61:320-6

Aimaretti G, Ambrosio MR, Di Somma C, Gasperi M, Cannavo S, Scaroni C, Fusco A, Del Monte P, De Menis E, Faustini-Fustini M, Grimaldi F, Logoluso F, Razzore P, Rovere S, Benvenga S, Degli Uberti EC, De Marinis L, Lombardi G, Mantero F, Martino E, Giordano G, Ghigo E (2005) Residual pituitary function after brain injury-induced hypopituitarism: a prospective 12-month study. *J Clin Endocrinol Metab* 90:6085-92

Altman R, Pruzanski W (1961) Post-traumatic hypopituitarism. Anterior pituitary insufficiency following skull fracture. *Ann Intern Med* 55:149-54

Avlonitis VS, Fisher AJ, Kirby JA, Dark JH (2003) Pulmonary transplantation: the role of brain death in donor lung injury. *Transplantation* 75:1928-33

Behan LA, Phillips J, Thompson CJ, Agha A (2008) Neuroendocrine disorders after traumatic brain injury. *J Neurol Neurosurg Psychiatry* 79:753-9

Benvenga S, Campenni A, Ruggeri RM, Trimarchi F (2000) Clinical review 113: Hypopituitarism secondary to head trauma. *J Clin Endocrinol Metab* 85:1353-61

Bettendorf M, Schmidt KG, Grulich-Henn J, Ulmer HE, Heinrich UE (2000) Tri-iodothyronine treatment in children after cardiac surgery: a double-blind, randomised, placebo-controlled study. *Lancet* 356:529-34

Bittner HB, Kendall SW, Chen EP, Van Trigt P (1995) Endocrine changes and metabolic responses in a validated canine brain death model. *J Crit Care* 10:56-63

Bondanelli M, De Marinis L, Ambrosio MR, Monesi M, Valle D, Zatelli MC, Fusco A, Bianchi A, Farneti M, degli Uberti EC (2004) Occurrence of pituitary dysfunction following traumatic brain injury. *J Neurotrauma* 21:685-96

Bondanelli M, Ambrosio MR, Zatelli MC, De Marinis L, degli Uberti EC (2005) Hypopituitarism after traumatic brain injury. *Eur J Endocrinol* 152:679-91

Bondanelli M, Ambrosio MR, Onofri A, Bergonzoni A, Lavezzi S, Zatelli MC, Valle D, Basaglia N, degli Uberti EC (2006) Predictive value of circulating insulin-like growth factor I levels in ischemic stroke outcome. *J Clin Endocrinol Metab* 91:3928-34

Boughey JC, Yost MJ, Bynoe RP (2004) Diabetes insipidus in the head-injured patient. *Am Surg* 70:500-3

Carroll PV, Christ ER, Bengtsson BA, Carlsson L, Christiansen JS, Clemmons D, Hintz R, Ho K, Laron Z, Sizonenko P, Sonksen PH, Tanaka T, Thorne M (1998) Growth hormone deficiency in adulthood and the effects of growth hormone replacement: a review. Growth Hormone Research Society Scientific Committee. *J Clin Endocrinol Metab* 83:382-95

Casanueva FF, Ghigo E, Popovic V (2004) Hypopituitarism following traumatic brain injury (TBI): a guideline decalogue. *J Endocrinol Invest* 27:793-5

Chamorro C, Falcon JA, Michelena JC (2009) Controversial points in organ donor management. *Transplant Proc* 41:3473-5

Chen EP, Bittner HB, Kendall SW, Van Trigt P (1996) Hormonal and hemodynamic changes in a validated animal model of brain death. *Crit Care Med* 24:1352-9

Chen JM, Cullinane S, Spanier TB, Artrip JH, John R, Edwards NM, Oz MC, Landry DW (1999) Vasopressin deficiency and pressor hypersensitivity in hemodynamically unstable organ donors. *Circulation* 100:II244-6

Chiolero R, Berger M (1994) Endocrine response to brain injury. *New Horiz* 2:432-42

Corneli G, Ghigo E, Aimaretti G (2007) Managing patients with hypopituitarism after traumatic brain injury. *Curr Opin Endocrinol Diabetes Obes* 14:301-5

Cyran E. (1918). *Hypophysenschädigung durch Schädelbasisfraktur.* , vol. 44, 1261.

Cytowic RE, Smith A, Stump DA (1986) Transient amenorrhea after closed head trauma. *N Engl J Med* 314:715

Daniel PM, Prichard MM, Treip CS (1959) Traumatic infarction of the anterior lobe of the pituitary gland. *Lancet* 2:927-31

Deijen JB, de Boer H, Blok GJ, van der Veen EA (1996) Cognitive impairments and mood disturbances in growth hormone deficient men. *Psychoneuroendocrinology* 21:313-22

Dimopoulou I, Tsagarakis S, Theodorakopoulou M, Douka E, Zervou M, Kouyialis AT, Thalassinos N, Roussos C (2004) Endocrine abnormalities in critical care patients with moderate-to-severe head trauma: incidence, pattern and predisposing factors. *Intensive Care Med* 30:1051-7

Edwards OM, Clark JD (1986) Post-traumatic hypopituitarism. Six cases and a review of the literature. *Medicine (Baltimore)* 65:281-90

Fisher AJ, Donnelly SC, Hirani N, Burdick MD, Strieter RM, Dark JH, Corris PA (1999) Enhanced pulmonary inflammation in organ donors following fatal non-traumatic brain injury. *Lancet* 353:1412-3

Follette DM, Rudich SM, Babcock WD (1998) Improved oxygenation and increased lung donor recovery with high-dose steroid administration after brain death. *J Heart Lung Transplant* 17:423-9

Ghigo E, Aimaretti G, Arvat E, Camanni F (2001) Growth hormone-releasing hormone combined with arginine or growth hormone secretagogues for the diagnosis of growth hormone deficiency in adults. *Endocrine* 15:29-38

Goarin JP, Cohen S, Riou B, Jacquens Y, Guesde R, Le Bret F, Aurengo A, Coriat P (1996) The effects of triiodothyronine on hemodynamic status and cardiac function in potential heart donors. *Anesth Analg* 83:41-7

Gordon AC, Russell JA, Walley KR, Singer J, Ayers D, Storms MM, Holmes CL, Hebert PC, Cooper DJ, Mehta S, Granton JT, Cook DJ, Presneill JJ (2010) The effects of vasopressin on acute kidney injury in septic shock. *Intensive Care Med* 36:83-91

Gramm HJ, Meinhold H, Bickel U, Zimmermann J, von Hammerstein B, Keller F, Dennhardt R, Voigt K (1992) Acute endocrine failure after brain death? *Transplantation* 54:851-7

Guesde R, Barrou B, Leblanc I, Ourahma S, Goarin JP, Coriat P, Riou B (1998) Administration of desmopressin in brain-dead donors and renal function in kidney recipients. *Lancet* 352:1178-81

Hartman ML, Crowe BJ, Biller BM, Ho KK, Clemmons DR, Chipman JJ (2002) Which patients do not require a GH stimulation test for the diagnosis of adult GH deficiency? *J Clin Endocrinol Metab* 87:477-85

Hing AJ, Hicks M, Garlick SR, Gao L, Kesteven SH, Faddy SC, Wilson MK, Feneley MP, Macdonald PS (2007) The effects of hormone resuscitation on cardiac function and hemodynamics in a porcine brain-dead organ donor model. *Am J Transplant* 7:809-17

Howlett TA, Keogh AM, Perry L, Touzel R, Rees LH (1989) Anterior and posterior pituitary function in brain-stem-dead donors. A possible role for hormonal replacement therapy. *Transplantation* 47:828-34

http://www.ccdt:ca/english/home.html Aa. Canidian Council for Donation and Transplantation. dec 2010

Ishikawa T, Michiue T, Quan L, Zhao D, Komatsu A, Bessho Y, Maeda H (2009) Morphological and functional alterations in the adenohypophysis in cases of brain death. *Leg Med (Tokyo)* 11 Suppl 1:S234-7

Kaufman HH, Timberlake G, Voelker J, Pait TG (1993) Medical complications of head injury. *Med Clin North Am* 77:43-60

Keegan M.T. KEW, and D.B. Coursin. (2009). *An update on ICU management of potential organ donor,*

Kelly DF, Gonzalo IT, Cohan P, Berman N, Swerdloff R, Wang C (2000) Hypopituitarism following traumatic brain injury and aneurysmal subarachnoid hemorrhage: a preliminary report. *J Neurosurg* 93:743-52

Kornblum RN, Fisher RS (1969) Pituitary lesions in craniocerebral injuries. *Arch Pathol* 88:242-8

Kotsch K, Ulrich F, Reutzel-Selke A, Pascher A, Faber W, Warnick P, Hoffman S, Francuski M, Kunert C, Kuecuek O, Schumacher G, Wesslau C, Lun A, Kohler S, Weiss S, Tullius SG, Neuhaus P, Pratschke J (2008) Methylprednisolone therapy in deceased donors reduces inflammation in the donor liver and improves outcome after liver transplantation: a prospective randomized controlled trial. *Ann Surg* 248:1042-50

Kreitschmann-Andermahr I, Hoff C, Saller B, Niggemeier S, Pruemper S, Hutter BO, Rohde V, Gressner A, Matern S, Gilsbach JM (2004) Prevalence of pituitary deficiency in patients after aneurysmal subarachnoid hemorrhage. *J Clin Endocrinol Metab* 89:4986-92

Kreutzer JS, Seel RT, Gourley E (2001) The prevalence and symptom rates of depression after traumatic brain injury: a comprehensive examination. *Brain Inj* 15:563-76

Kusanagi H, Kogure K, Teramoto A (2000) Pituitary insufficiency after penetrating injury to the sella turcica. *J Nippon Med Sch* 67:130-3

LaChapelle DL, Finlayson MA (1998) An evaluation of subjective and objective measures of fatigue in patients with brain injury and healthy controls. *Brain Inj* 12:649-59

Lamberts SW, de Herder WW, van der Lely AJ (1998) Pituitary insufficiency. *Lancet* 352:127-34

Leon-Carrion J, De Serdio-Arias ML, Cabezas FM, Roldan JM, Dominguez-Morales R, Martin JM, Sanchez MA (2001) Neurobehavioural and cognitive profile of traumatic brain injury patients at risk for depression and suicide. *Brain Inj* 15:175-81

Lieberman SA, Oberoi AL, Gilkison CR, Masel BE, Urban RJ (2001) Prevalence of neuroendocrine dysfunction in patients recovering from traumatic brain injury. *J Clin Endocrinol Metab* 86:2752-6

Lissett CA SS. (1996). *Hypopituitarism,*

Mascia L, Bosma K, Pasero D, Galli T, Cortese G, Donadio P, Bosco R (2006) Ventilatory and hemodynamic management of potential organ donors: an observational survey. *Crit Care Med* 34:321-7; quiz 8

Mascia L, Mastromauro I, Viberti S, Vincenzi M, Zanello M (2009) Management to optimize organ procurement in brain dead donors. *Minerva Anestesiol* 75:125-33

Mascia L, Pasero D, Slutsky AS, Arguis MJ, Berardino M, Grasso S, Munari M, Boifava S, Cornara G, Della Corte F, Vivaldi N, Malacarne P, Del Gaudio P, Livigni S, Zavala E, Filippini C, Martin EL, Donadio PP, Mastromauro I, Ranieri VM (2010) Effect of a lung protective strategy for organ donors on eligibility and availability of lungs for transplantation: a randomized controlled trial. *JAMA* 304:2620-7

Mutlu GM, Factor P (2004) Role of vasopressin in the management of septic shock. *Intensive Care Med* 30:1276-91

Novitzky D, Cooper DK, Morrell D, Isaacs S (1988) Change from aerobic to anaerobic metabolism after brain death, and reversal following triiodothyronine therapy. *Transplantation* 45:32-6

Novitzky D, Cooper DK, Chaffin JS, Greer AE, DeBault LE, Zuhdi N (1990) Improved cardiac allograft function following triiodothyronine therapy to both donor and recipient. *Transplantation* 49:311-6

Novitzky D, Cooper DK, Rosendale JD, Kauffman HM (2006) Hormonal therapy of the brain-dead organ donor: experimental and clinical studies. *Transplantation* 82:1396-401

Pennefather SH, Bullock RE, Mantle D, Dark JH (1995) Use of low dose arginine vasopressin to support brain-dead organ donors. *Transplantation* 59:58-62

Rosendale JD, Chabalewski FL, McBride MA, Garrity ER, Rosengard BR, Delmonico FL, Kauffman HM (2002) Increased transplanted organs from the use of a standardized donor management protocol. *Am J Transplant* 2:761-8

Rosendale JD, Kauffman HM, McBride MA, Chabalewski FL, Zaroff JG, Garrity ER, Delmonico FL, Rosengard BR (2003a) Hormonal resuscitation yields more transplanted hearts, with improved early function. *Transplantation* 75:1336-41

Rosendale JD, Kauffman HM, McBride MA, Chabalewski FL, Zaroff JG, Garrity ER, Delmonico FL, Rosengard BR (2003b) Aggressive pharmacologic donor management results in more transplanted organs. *Transplantation* 75:482-7

Rosengard BR, Feng S, Alfrey EJ, Zaroff JG, Emond JC, Henry ML, Garrity ER, Roberts JP, Wynn JJ, Metzger RA, Freeman RB, Port FK, Merion RM, Love RB, Busuttil RW, Delmonico FL (2002) Report of the Crystal City meeting to maximize the use of organs recovered from the cadaver donor. *Am J Transplant* 2:701-11

Rostron AJ, Avlonitis VS, Cork DM, Grenade DS, Kirby JA, Dark JH (2008) Hemodynamic resuscitation with arginine vasopressin reduces lung injury after brain death in the transplant donor. *Transplantation* 85:597-606

Salim A, Vassiliu P, Velmahos GC, Sava J, Murray JA, Belzberg H, Asensio JA, Demetriades D (2001) The role of thyroid hormone administration in potential organ donors. *Arch Surg* 136:1377-80

Salim A, Martin M, Brown C, Belzberg H, Rhee P, Demetriades D (2006) Complications of brain death: frequency and impact on organ retrieval. *Am Surg* 72:377-81

Schneider HJ, Rovere S, Corneli G, Croce CG, Gasco V, Ruda R, Grottoli S, Stalla GK, Soffietti R, Ghigo E, Aimaretti G (2006) Endocrine dysfunction in patients operated on for non-pituitary intracranial tumors. *Eur J Endocrinol* 155:559-66

Schneider HJ, Kreitschmann-Andermahr I, Ghigo E, Stalla GK, Agha A (2007) Hypothalamopituitary dysfunction following traumatic brain injury and aneurysmal subarachnoid hemorrhage: a systematic review. *JAMA* 298:1429-38

Smith M (2004) Physiologic changes during brain stem death--lessons for management of the organ donor. *J Heart Lung Transplant* 23:S217-22

Ullah S, Zabala L, Watkins B, Schmitz ML (2006) Cardiac organ donor management. *Perfusion* 21:93-8

Van den Berghe G, de Zegher F (1996) Anterior pituitary function during critical illness and dopamine treatment. *Crit Care Med* 24:1580-90

Van den Berghe G, de Zegher F, Bouillon R (1998) The somatotrophic axis in critical illness: effects of growth hormone secretagogues. *Growth Horm IGF Res* 8 Suppl B:153-5

Venkateswaran RV, Dronavalli V, Lambert PA, Steeds RP, Wilson IC, Thompson RD, Mascaro JG, Bonser RS (2009a) The proinflammatory environment in potential heart and lung donors: prevalence and impact of donor management and hormonal therapy. *Transplantation* 88:582-8

Venkateswaran RV, Steeds RP, Quinn DW, Nightingale P, Wilson IC, Mascaro JG, Thompson RD, Townend JN, Bonser RS (2009b) The haemodynamic effects of adjunctive hormone therapy in potential heart donors: a prospective randomized double-blind factorially designed controlled trial. *Eur Heart J* 30:1771-80

Wheeldon DR, Potter CD, Oduro A, Wallwork J, Large SR (1995) Transforming the "unacceptable" donor: outcomes from the adoption of a standardized donor management technique. *J Heart Lung Transplant* 14:734-42

Wong MF, Chin NM, Lew TW (1998) Diabetes insipidus in neurosurgical patients. *Ann Acad Med Singapore* 27:340-3

Wood KE, Becker BN, McCartney JG, D'Alessandro AM, Coursin DB (2004) Care of the potential organ donor. *N Engl J Med* 351:2730-9

Yoshioka T, Sugimoto H, Uenishi M, Sakamoto T, Sadamitsu D, Sakano T, Sugimoto T (1986) Prolonged hemodynamic maintenance by the combined administration of vasopressin and epinephrine in brain death: a clinical study. *Neurosurgery* 18:565-7

Yuan XQ, Wade CE (1991) Neuroendocrine abnormalities in patients with traumatic brain injury. *Front Neuroendocrinol* 12:209-30

Zaroff JG, Rosengard BR, Armstrong WF, Babcock WD, D'Alessandro A, Dec GW, Edwards NM, Higgins RS, Jeevanandum V, Kauffman M, Kirklin JK, Large SR, Marelli D, Peterson TS, Ring WS, Robbins RC, Russell SD, Taylor DO, Van Bakel A, Wallwork J, Young JB (2002) Consensus conference report: maximizing use of organs recovered from the cadaver donor: cardiac recommendations, March 28-29, 2001, Crystal City, Va. *Circulation* 106:836-41

4

Nephrogenic Diabetes Insipidus – The Novelly Potential Therapeutic Drugs

Jessica Y.S. Chu and Billy K.C. Chow
School of Biological Sciences, The University of Hong Kong, Hong Kong, China

1. Introduction

Water reabsorption in the kidney represents a critical physiological event in the maintenance of body water homeostasis. This highly regulated process relies largely on the antidiuretic hormone, vasopressin (VP), and on the VP-sensitive aquaporin-2 (AQP2) water channel that is expressed in the principal cells of kidney collecting duct. Under normal condition, AQP2 resides in the intracellular vesicles of the principal cells. Apical plasma membrane facing the primary urine of these cells therefore contains only low amounts of water channels and is relatively water impermeable. When there is increased plasma osmolality or hypovolemia, VP released from the neurohypophysis binds to its cognate VP type 2 receptor (V2R) that is expressed on the basolateral membrane of the collecting duct principal cells. This elevates intracellular cAMP concentration and promotes protein kinase A (PKA) activity that lead to phosphorylation of AQP2 at Ser^{256} (Christensen et al., 2000), as well as phosphorylation of Rho at Ser^{188} (Tamma et al., 2001; Tamma et al., 2003). AQP2 phosphorylation allows their redistribution from intracellular location to apical plasma membrane, whereas Rho phosphorylation results in a subsequent attenuation of Rho activity that favors the depolymerization of F-actin (Tamma et al., 2001; Tamma et al., 2003). This latter action allows removal of the cytoskeleton barrier that blocks the passage of AQP2 to the plasma membrane. Therefore, with the presence of AQP2 on the apical membrane of principal cells, a strong increase of water permeability of this membrane compartment is resulted. This allows acceleration of water reabsorption from primary urine, thus compensating for body water loss during hypovolemic or hypernatremic state.

Defects in the function of V2R and/or in AQP2 cell surface expression (known as nephrogenic diabetes insipidus or NDI) may perpetuate alteration of the biological boundaries that maintain plasma osmolality within a well defined, but very narrow physiological range. Patients having which are unable to concentrate their urine despite normal or elevated plasma concentrations of VP, thereby at the risk of hypernatremic dehydration and having manifestations including polyuria, polydipsia, hyposthenuria, recurrent episodes of dehydration, fever, and even growth failure. Despite the molecular defects underlying this disorder has now been revealed and has enabled a successful diagnosis, no cure is currently exists for NDI. Instead, this condition is managed by restriction in sodium intake combined with the administration of hydrochlorothiazide diuretics to reduce urine output, which might nonetheless lead to hypovolemia and hypokalemia (Blanchard et al., 2008). The search for more effective therapeutic strategies for NDI therefore is needed. Consistent with this notion, identifying V2R-independent mechanisms that regulate AQP2 trafficking could definitely be beneficial for the exploration of novel therapeutic strategies in the treatment of NDI, as this disorder is most commonly resulted from mutations in V2R gene (~90%).

2. Factors involved in V2R-independent cAMP pathway

2.1 Secretin

Apart from VP, various other physiological factors that modulate AQP2 cell-surface localization via the cAMP pathway have been uncovered. One of such factors is secretin (SCT), a 27-amino acid peptide hormone that modulates transepithelial movement of water and electrolyte in varies tissues. Clinically, serum concentration of SCT was found to increase significantly in hemodialysis patients (Grekas et al., 1984) and in patients with chronic renal failure (Hansky, 1979) in comparison to controls, indicating that the peptide might be associated with clinical-pathological status of the kidney. Morphologically, the kidneys of SCT receptor (SCTR)-deficient ($SCTR^{-/-}$) mice were abnormal, characterized by increased mesangial area, enlarged urinary space, and frequent tubular dilation and hypertrophy in the collecting tubules of the medullary region (Chu et al., 2007), suggesting they might have altered water absorption and filtration processes. Consistent with this notion, in vitro treatment of SCT was found to induce a dose-dependent increase in AQP2 expression on the plasma membrane and a dose-dependent decrease in AQP2 expression in the intracellular vesicles (Cheng et al., 2009; Chu et al., 2007). This induced translocation of AQP2 was mediated via a cAMP/PKA-dependent pathway (Cheng et al., 2009), and was shown to be absent in the medullary tubules isolated from $SCTR^{-/-}$ (Chu et al., 2007), hence indicating that the peptide induces the movement of AQP2 upon binding with its receptor. Because SCT can be released from the hypothalamo-pituitary axis (Chu et al., 2009), and that $SCTR^{-/-}$ mice exhibit normal levels of plasma VP as well as V2R in their kidney when compared to their wild-type littermates (Chu et al., 2007), these data collectively indicated a role of SCT in VP-independent stimulation of the expression and movement of AQP2s in the kidney. This concept was further substantiated by the fact that Charlton *et al.* (Charlton et al., 1986) was able to show an antidiuretic effect of SCT as potent as VP in homozygous VP-deficient Brattleboro rats, whereas Chu *et al.* (Chu et al., 2007) detected an altered response in AQP2 movement to the plasma membrane during hyperosmolality in $SCTR^{-/-}$ mice. Therefore, all these data suggested that SCT could also be of great interest to the NDI community as it shows a direction of study for developing therapies to treat NDI that are independent of the VP pathway.

2.2 Calcitonin

The second factor that has been proven to by-pass the VP-dependent simulation of AQP2 translocation via the cAMP pathway is calcitonin, which is a 32-amino acid peptide hormone that was found to have its plasma concentration increase in acute and chronic renal failure (Ardaillou, 1975; Ardaillou et al., 1975). Early work by de Rouffignac and Elalouf (de Rouffignac and Elalouf, 1983) proposed that the peptide hormone could exert a VP-like effect on electrolyte transport by the thick ascending limb and/or on the water permeability of the cortical collecting ducts. This observation has recently been confirmed by another group showing a stimulation of the membrane accumulation of AQP2 by calcitonin in the LLC-PK1 cells as well as in the cortical collecting ducts on rat kidney slices (Bouley et al., 2011). Using osmotic pumps implanted into VP-deficient Brattleboro rats, they also discovered that calcitonin-treated rats urinate less, and their urine was more concentrated than in the control group, indicating that the peptide could play a direct role in the urinary concentrating mechanism. Additional studies therefore are required to further examining the antidiuretic effect of calcitonin as well as to determine whether this peptide might be beneficial to patients suffering from X-linked NDI.

3. Factors involved in nitric oxide/cGMP pathway

Together with the canonical cAMP-induced pathway, the nitric oxide (NO)/cGMP signaling pathway has been shown to play a role in AQP2 trafficking/expression, prompting investigation of this signaling pathway as a means to develop alternative therapies for treatment of NDI. NO is a very active free radical that produced enzymatically by one of the three (i.e. endothelial, neuronal, and inducible) intracellularly located nitric oxide synthase (NOS) isoforms that convert L-arginine to citrulline. It plays an important role in overall excretory function of the kidney (Majid and Navar, 2001) and is involved in the development of kidney dysfunction in several diseases, including diabetes and hypertension (Palm et al., 2009). In the classical NO signaling pathway, NO acts on the soluble guanylyl cyclase (GC), leading to an increased production of the second messenger cyclic guanosine monophosphate (cGMP). This then influences various intracellular functions via activation of the protein kinase G. cGMP, however, can also affects cAMP signals (Stangherlin et al., 2011) as well as PKA activity (Yamada et al., 2006), which are both mediated via cGMP-regulated phosphodiesterases (PDEs) (Stangherlin et al., 2011). By binding to the regulatory GAF-B domain at the N-terminus of PDE2, cGMP potently activates its cAMP hydrolyzing activity (Martinez et al., 2002). Through such a regulatory mechanism, stimuli that elevate cGMP could attenuate cAMP-dependent signaling pathway (Michie et al., 1996). Conversely, cGMP could also act effectively as a competitive inhibitor of PDE3 cAMP-degrading activity (Shakur et al., 2001). As a consequence, PDE3 provides a means by which an increase in cGMP may lead to an increase in cAMP.

The components of the NO-cGMP signaling pathway were found to be expressed throughout the kidney (Bachmann et al., 1995; Tojo et al., 1994; Ujiie et al., 1994), supporting the notion that the NO-cGMP signaling pathway plays a key role in renal physiology, including fluid transport. In consistent with this notion, Bouley *et al.* (Bouley et al., 2000) found that AQP2 insertion could be accomplished by the activation of the cGMP-dependent pathway. They showed that NO donors, such as sodium nitroprusside and NONOate, as well as the NOS substrate L-arginine, appeared to induce AQP2 translocation from intracellular vesicles to the apical membrane by increasing cGMP levels in rat kidney slices and AQP2-transfected LLC-PK1 cells. Similarly, another study by Martin *et al.* (Martin et al., 2002) showed that water deprivation induced the expression of endothelial NOS and neuronal NOS in the outer medulla as well as both the outer medulla and the papilla, respectively, which could be subsequently decreased by water loading. Other evidence further supporting the idea that NO-cGMP plays a role in water homeostatic mechanisms came from the fact that 1) VP specifically increases neuronal NOS expression levels in the renal outer medulla and papilla (Martin et al., 2002), 2) an increased expression of AQP2 within the kidneys of cirrhotic rats was found to correlate with the increasing activities of NOS (Jun et al., 2010), and 3) simultaneous disruption of all three NOS isoforms led to reduce membranous AQP2 expression associated with tubuloglomerular lesion formation, as well as marked hypotonic polyuria, polydipsia, and renal unresponsiveness to VP (Morishita et al., 2005), all of which are characteristics consistent with NDI. Thus, AQP2 expression and trafficking, which is chiefly regulated by VP, may be additionally stimulated by NO-cGMP activity.

3.1 Atrial Natriuretic Peptide (ANP)

ANP is a 28-amino acid peptide that is well established to activate membrane-bound GC and modulates cellular functions via the intracellular second messenger cGMP. Consistent with this, studies have provided evidence for stimulation of cGMP production in various renal tubule segments in response to ANP (Nonoguchi et al., 1987; Takeda et al., 1986) and for the expression of the cGMP-coupled ANP receptor in these segments (Terada et al., 1991). However, the effect of ANP (through an increase in cGMP) on sodium and fluid transport in the collecting duct is still controversial. Some earlier studies showed that it decreases both sodium reabsorption and vasopressin-induced water transport in collecting ducts (Dillingham and Anderson, 1986; Nonoguchi et al., 1988; Nonoguchi et al., 1989), whereas later studies do not confirm these inhibitory effects (Bouley et al., 2000; Rouch et al., 1991). This might probably due to the fact that ANP has a biphasic effects on renal water reabsorption process. Wang *et al.* (Wang et al., 2006) in a more recent study demonstrated that ANP infusion (0.5 μg/kg/min) evoked a transient (peak at 10 min) but significant diuresis (~5 fold), with no changes in GFR as well as the subcellular localization of AQP2, followed by a decrease in water excretion, accompanied by a marked increase in apical targeting of AQP2, 90 min after infusion. This effect of ANP on AQP2 was further confirmed by both Bouley *et al.* (Bouley et al., 2000) and Wang *et al.* (Wang et al., 2006) in *in-vitro* studies using AQP2-expressing LLC-PK1 cells and AQP2-transfected HEK 293 cells, respectively. The former group also postulated that Ser^{256} of AQP2 is the target motif for stimulation by ANF. Because there are marked changes in water excretion seen in response to acute (10 min) and subacute (90 min) ANP treatment, a detail understanding of the underlying mechanisms that governs these processes is needed before considering whether ANP could be use as a therapeutic strategy for the treatment of NDI.

3.2 Sildenafil citrate (Viagra)

The use of Viagra, a selective PDE5 inhibitor, as potential therapeutic agents for NDI has been described. Bouley *et al.* (Bouley et al., 2005) found that 45-min exposure of AQP2-transfected LLC-PK1 cells to either Viagra or 4-{[3',4'-methylene-dioxybenzyl]amino}-6-methoxyquinazoline elevates intracellular cGMP levels and results in the plasma membrane accumulation of AQP2. They also demonstrated that exposure to PDE5 inhibitors for 60 min could induce an apical accumulation of AQP2 in renal medullary collecting duct principal cells both in tissue slices incubated *in-vitro* as well as *in-vivo* after intravenous injection of Viagra into rats. While Viagra has been successfully used in the clinical treatment of erectile dysfunction and that research data suggested that PDE inhibition by this drug may offer a promising approach for X-linked NDI therapy, further studies are needed in order to determine whether prolonged viagra or cGMP inhibition, or a combined therapeutic approach, can improve water reabsorption in patients suffering from NDI who may express variable amounts of AQP2 in their principal cells.

4. Factors involved in AQP2 endocytosis and exocytosis

About 10% of NDI cases are associated with AQP2 mutations rather than with defects of V2R signalling. Interestingly, most mutations identified in the AQP2 gene in NDI are manifested as mis-routing errors rather than as structural defects that affect their ability in conducting water across the membrane. Some of these mutations, including L22V, L28P, A47V, V71M, T126M, A147T, V168M, P185A, R187C, E258K, and P262L have been characterized in Xenopus oocytes, yeast, and/or mammalian cells, and have been shown to have impaired folding, resulting in recognition by the endoplasmic reticulum (ER) quality control machinery, ubiquitination, and degradation by the 26S proteasome (Boccalandro et al., 2004; de Mattia et al., 2004; Deen et al., 1995; Kamsteeg et al., 2008; Kamsteeg et al., 2009; Levin et al., 2001; Marr et al., 2002; Mulders et al., 1997; Tamarappoo and Verkman, 1998). However, these AQP2 mutants are found to be intrinsically functional water channels when being characterized. In light of the fact that AQP2 rapidly and constitutively recycle between the plasma membrane and intracellular vesicles, even in the absence of any stimulation (Lu et al., 2004), and that channel gating of AQP2 is independent of the membrane insertion/trafficking process (Moeller et al., 2009), therapeutic strategies for NDI caused by AQP2 mutation could be bought either by agents that stimulate AQP2 excytosis, or agents that causes a reduction in the rate of AQP2 endocytosis. Consistent with this notion, an extensive accumulation of AQP2 at the cell surface was successfully accomplished within 30 min after inhibition of endocytosis by treatment with cholesterol-depleting drug, methyl-β-cyclodextrin (Lu et al., 2004; Russo et al., 2006), which prevents the formation and budding of clathrin-coated pits. This implies that while we are looking for V2R-independent signalling pathways to induce an increase translocation of AQP2 to the cell surface, any agent that inhibits the endocytosis of intrinsically functional AQP2 mutant may consequently represent an alternative strategy for therapeutic intervention in NDI.

4.1 Chemical chaperones

Chemical chaperones, which are protein-folding enhancers, have already been shown to act as the potential therapeutic agents for the control of many of the protein conformational diseases, including Alzheimer's disease (Evans et al., 2006), Prion's disease (Tatzelt et al., 1996), and cystic fibrosis (Brown et al., 1996). As most of the AQP2 mutants are associated with defect in folding, leading to their accumulation within intracellular compartment, an observation of the corrective effect of chemical chaperones on defective AQP2 trafficking in NDI is therefore not peculiar. In this regards, Tamarappoo and Verkman (Tamarappoo and Verkman, 1998) found that incubating chemical chaperones, including glycerol, trimethylamine oxide (TMAO), and dimethyl sulfoxide (DMSO), to AQP2 mutant-expressing cells could produced a nearly complete redistribution of the mutants from endoplasmic reticulum to membrane/endosome fractions, achieving functional correction of the processing defect. Similarly, another group also showed that Hsp90 inhibitor, 17-allylamino-17-demethoxygeldanamycin (17-AAG), produced partial correction of the defective AQP2 cellular processing in transfected kidney cells (Yang et al., 2009). They also observed an increase urine osmolality in AQP2 mutant-expressing mice when intraperitoneally injected with 17-AAG, demonstrating a function of this chemical chaperones in improving urinary concentrating function. As 17-AAG is currently in phase 2 clinical trials for several cancer targets (Pacey et al., 2010), and that recent data showing promising therapeutic activity of the compound (Kurashina et al., 2009; Yao et al., 2010), 17-AAG or other chemical chaperones may be useful for therapy of some forms of NDI.

4.2 Simvastatin

Simvastatin, a family of 3-hydroxy-3-methylglutaryl coenzyme A reductase inhibitors, was originally developed as therapeutic agents for reducing cholesterol and hence the prevention and treatment of cardiovascular diseases (O'Driscoll et al., 1997; Olsson et al., 2011). Recent studies, however, have revealed more of its pleiotropic effects including cognition enhancement (Douma et al., 2011), anti-inflammation (Nezic et al., 2009; Zhang et al., 2011), and anti-cancer activity (Miller et al., 2011). More interestingly, studies *in-vitro* also suggested that it could inhibit the endocytosis of proteins in proximal tubule cells via its inhibitory effects on prenylation and thereby the function of one or more GTP-binding proteins (Sidaway et al., 2004), suggesting a similar role of its in regulating AQP2 membrane presentation. Consistent with this notion, simvastatin was shown to induces AQP2 membrane accumulation via its inhibitory effect on AQP2 endocytosis, which was independent of cAMP/PKA activation and also Ser^{256} phosphorylation of AQP2 (Li et al., 2011). These authors also found that intraperitoneal injection of simvastatin to VP-deficient Brattleboro rats resulted in decreased urinary volume with simultaneously increased urinary osmolality, hence its effect on renal water reabsorption and urinary concentration. Therefore, even though the total reduction of urine output may seem to be modest with simvastatin-treated animals, simvastatin treatment might still be significant for NDI patients who may produce up to 10-15 liters of urine each day.

Factors involved in V2R-independent cAMP pathway
Secretin
Calcitonin
Factors involved in nitric oxide/cGMP pathway
Atrial natriuretic peptide
Sildenafil citrate (Viagra) and other PDE inhibitors
Factors involved in AQP2 endocytosis and exocytosis
Chemical chaperones
• Glycerol
• Trimethylamine oxide (TMAO)
• Dimethyl sulfoxide (DMSO)
• Hsp90 inhibitor 17-allylamino-17-demethoxygeldanamycin (17-AAG)
Cholesterol-depleting drug
• Methyl-β-cyclodextrin
• Simvastatin

Table 1. List of the potential therapeutic drugs that increase membrane presentation of AQP2.

5. Conclusion

Recent advances in the understanding of AQP2 recycling and the signaling pathways that lead to the membrane accumulation of AQP2 in renal collecting tubular principal cells have opened up several possible strategies for inducing this process in the absence of conventional VP signaling via its receptor, which is defective in X-linked NDI (Table 1). Some of these strategies are potential to serve as basis for the development of novel therapies that may ultimately improve life quality of NDI patients. Therefore, identifying analogs of these potential agents with reduced cytoxicity and also improved pharmacological properties are necessary for preclinical development. Depending on the nature of the defect leading to this disorder, it is very likely that a combination of different approaches, directed by the basic research endeavors that are ongoing in many labs, will be needed to achieve a positive clinical outcome.

6. Acknowledgment

The authors thank the research supported by the HK government RGC grant HKU7501/05 M and HKU7384/04 M to BKCC.

7. References

Ardaillou, R., 1975. Kidney and calcitonin. Nephron. 15, 250-60.

Ardaillou, R., Beaufils, M., Nivez, M.P., Isaac, R., Mayaud, C., Sraer, J.D., 1975. Increased plasma calcitonin in early acute renal failure. Clin Sci Mol Med. 49, 301-4.

Bachmann, S., Bosse, H.M., Mundel, P., 1995. Topography of nitric oxide synthesis by localizing constitutive NO synthases in mammalian kidney. Am J Physiol. 268, F885-98.

Blanchard, A., Vargas-Poussou, R., Peyrard, S., Mogenet, A., Baudouin, V., Boudailliez, B., Charbit, M., Deschesnes, G., Ezzhair, N., Loirat, C., Macher, M.A., Niaudet, P., Azizi, M., 2008. Effect of hydrochlorothiazide on urinary calcium excretion in dent disease: an uncontrolled trial. Am J Kidney Dis. 52, 1084-95.

Boccalandro, C., De Mattia, F., Guo, D.C., Xue, L., Orlander, P., King, T.M., Gupta, P., Deen, P.M., Lavis, V.R., Milewicz, D.M., 2004. Characterization of an aquaporin-2 water channel gene mutation causing partial nephrogenic diabetes insipidus in a Mexican family: evidence of increased frequency of the mutation in the town of origin. J Am Soc Nephrol. 15, 1223-31.

Bouley, R., Breton, S., Sun, T., McLaughlin, M., Nsumu, N.N., Lin, H.Y., Ausiello, D.A., Brown, D., 2000. Nitric oxide and atrial natriuretic factor stimulate cGMP-dependent membrane insertion of aquaporin 2 in renal epithelial cells. J Clin Invest. 106, 1115-26.

Bouley, R., Pastor-Soler, N., Cohen, O., McLaughlin, M., Breton, S., Brown, D., 2005. Stimulation of AQP2 membrane insertion in renal epithelial cells in vitro and in vivo by the cGMP phosphodiesterase inhibitor sildenafil citrate (Viagra). Am J Physiol Renal Physiol. 288, F1103-12.

Bouley, R., Lu, H.A., Nunes, P., Da Silva, N., McLaughlin, M., Chen, Y., Brown, D., 2011. Calcitonin has a vasopressin-like effect on aquaporin-2 trafficking and urinary concentration. J Am Soc Nephrol. 22, 59-72.

Brown, C.R., Hong-Brown, L.Q., Biwersi, J., Verkman, A.S., Welch, W.J., 1996. Chemical chaperones correct the mutant phenotype of the delta F508 cystic fibrosis transmembrane conductance regulator protein. Cell Stress Chaperones. 1, 117-25.

Charlton, C.G., Quirion, R., Handelmann, G.E., Miller, R.L., Jensen, R.T., Finkel, M.S., O'Donohue, T.L., 1986. Secretin receptors in the rat kidney: adenylate cyclase activation and renal effects. Peptides. 7, 865-71.

Cheng, C.Y., Chu, J.Y., Chow, B.K., 2009. Vasopressin-independent mechanisms in controlling water homeostasis. J Mol Endocrinol. 43, 81-92.

Christensen, B.M., Zelenina, M., Aperia, A., Nielsen, S., 2000. Localization and regulation of PKA-phosphorylated AQP2 in response to V(2)-receptor agonist/antagonist treatment. Am J Physiol Renal Physiol. 278, F29-42.

Chu, J.Y., Chung, S.C., Lam, A.K., Tam, S., Chung, S.K., Chow, B.K., 2007. Phenotypes developed in secretin receptor-null mice indicated a role for secretin in regulating renal water reabsorption. Mol Cell Biol. 27, 2499-511.

Chu, J.Y., Lee, L.T., Lai, C.H., Vaudry, H., Chan, Y.S., Yung, W.H., Chow, B.K., 2009. Secretin as a neurohypophysial factor regulating body water homeostasis. Proc Natl Acad Sci U S A. 106, 15961-6.

de Mattia, F., Savelkoul, P.J., Bichet, D.G., Kamsteeg, E.J., Konings, I.B., Marr, N., Arthus, M.F., Lonergan, M., van Os, C.H., van der Sluijs, P., Robertson, G., Deen, P.M., 2004. A novel mechanism in recessive nephrogenic diabetes insipidus: wild-type aquaporin-2 rescues the apical membrane expression of intracellularly retained AQP2-P262L. Hum Mol Genet. 13, 3045-56.

de Rouffignac, C., Elalouf, J.M., 1983. Effects of calcitonin on the renal concentrating mechanism. Am J Physiol. 245, F506-11.

Deen, P.M., Croes, H., van Aubel, R.A., Ginsel, L.A., van Os, C.H., 1995. Water channels encoded by mutant aquaporin-2 genes in nephrogenic diabetes insipidus are impaired in their cellular routing. J Clin Invest. 95, 2291-6.

Dillingham, M.A., Anderson, R.J., 1986. Inhibition of vasopressin action by atrial natriuretic factor. Science. 231, 1572-3.

Douma, T.N., Borre, Y., Hendriksen, H., Olivier, B., Oosting, R.S., 2011. Simvastatin improves learning and memory in control but not in olfactory bulbectomized rats. Psychopharmacology (Berl).

Evans, C.G., Wisen, S., Gestwicki, J.E., 2006. Heat shock proteins 70 and 90 inhibit early stages of amyloid beta-(1-42) aggregation in vitro. J Biol Chem. 281, 33182-91.

Grekas, D.M., Raptis, S., Tourkantonis, A.A., 1984. Plasma secretin, pancreozymin, and somatostatin-like hormone in chronic renal failure patients. Uremia Invest. 8, 117-20.

Hansky, J., 1979. Effect of renal failure on gastrointestinal hormones. World J Surg. 3, 463-7.

Jun, D.W., Park, J.H., Park, Y.S., Kang, J.S., Kim, E.K., Kim, K.T., Son, B.K., Kim, S.H., Jo, Y.J., 2010. The role of nitric oxide in the expression of renal aquaporin 2 in a cirrhotic rat model: does an AVP-independent mechanism exist for the regulation of AQP2 expression? Dig Dis Sci. 55, 1296-304.

Kamsteeg, E.J., Savelkoul, P.J., Hendriks, G., Konings, I.B., Nivillac, N.M., Lagendijk, A.K., van der Sluijs, P., Deen, P.M., 2008. Missorting of the Aquaporin-2 mutant E258K to multivesicular bodies/lysosomes in dominant NDI is associated with its monoubiquitination and increased phosphorylation by PKC but is due to the loss of E258. Pflugers Arch. 455, 1041-54.

Kamsteeg, E.J., Stoffels, M., Tamma, G., Konings, I.B., Deen, P.M., 2009. Repulsion between Lys258 and upstream arginines explains the missorting of the AQP2 mutant p.Glu258Lys in nephrogenic diabetes insipidus. Hum Mutat. 30, 1387-96.

Kurashina, R., Ohyashiki, J.H., Kobayashi, C., Hamamura, R., Zhang, Y., Hirano, T., Ohyashiki, K., 2009. Anti-proliferative activity of heat shock protein (Hsp) 90 inhibitors via beta-catenin/TCF7L2 pathway in adult T cell leukemia cells. Cancer Lett. 284, 62-70.

Levin, M.H., Haggie, P.M., Vetrivel, L., Verkman, A.S., 2001. Diffusion in the endoplasmic reticulum of an aquaporin-2 mutant causing human nephrogenic diabetes insipidus. J Biol Chem. 276, 21331-6.

Li, W., Zhang, Y., Bouley, R., Chen, Y., Matsuzaki, T., Nunes, P., Hasler, U., Brown, D., Lu, H.A., 2011. Simvastatin Enhances Aquaporin 2 Surface Expression and Urinary Concentration in Vasopressin Deficient Brattleboro Rats through Modulation of Rho GTPase. Am J Physiol Renal Physiol.

Lu, H., Sun, T.X., Bouley, R., Blackburn, K., McLaughlin, M., Brown, D., 2004. Inhibition of endocytosis causes phosphorylation (S256)-independent plasma membrane accumulation of AQP2. Am J Physiol Renal Physiol. 286, F233-43.

Majid, D.S., Navar, L.G., 2001. Nitric oxide in the control of renal hemodynamics and excretory function. Am J Hypertens. 14, 74S-82S.

Marr, N., Bichet, D.G., Hoefs, S., Savelkoul, P.J., Konings, I.B., De Mattia, F., Graat, M.P., Arthus, M.F., Lonergan, M., Fujiwara, T.M., Knoers, N.V., Landau, D., Balfe, W.J., Oksche, A., Rosenthal, W., Muller, D., Van Os, C.H., Deen, P.M., 2002. Cell-biologic and functional analyses of five new Aquaporin-2 missense mutations that cause recessive nephrogenic diabetes insipidus. J Am Soc Nephrol. 13, 2267-77.

Martin, P.Y., Bianchi, M., Roger, F., Niksic, L., Feraille, E., 2002. Arginine vasopressin modulates expression of neuronal NOS in rat renal medulla. Am J Physiol Renal Physiol. 283, F559-68.

Martinez, S.E., Beavo, J.A., Hol, W.G., 2002. GAF domains: two-billion-year-old molecular switches that bind cyclic nucleotides. Mol Interv. 2, 317-23.

Michie, A.M., Lobban, M., Muller, T., Harnett, M.M., Houslay, M.D., 1996. Rapid regulation of PDE-2 and PDE-4 cyclic AMP phosphodiesterase activity following ligation of the T cell antigen receptor on thymocytes: analysis using the selective inhibitors erythro-9-(2-hydroxy-3-nonyl)-adenine (EHNA) and rolipram. Cell Signal. 8, 97-110.

Miller, T., Yang, F., Wise, C.E., Meng, F., Priester, S., Munshi, M.K., Guerrier, M., Dostal, D.E., Glaser, S.S., 2011. Simvastatin stimulates apoptosis in cholangiocarcinoma by inhibition of Rac1 activity. Dig Liver Dis. 43, 395-403.

Moeller, H.B., MacAulay, N., Knepper, M.A., Fenton, R.A., 2009. Role of multiple phosphorylation sites in the COOH-terminal tail of aquaporin-2 for water transport: evidence against channel gating. Am J Physiol Renal Physiol. 296, F649-57.

Morishita, T., Tsutsui, M., Shimokawa, H., Sabanai, K., Tasaki, H., Suda, O., Nakata, S., Tanimoto, A., Wang, K.Y., Ueta, Y., Sasaguri, Y., Nakashima, Y., Yanagihara, N., 2005. Nephrogenic diabetes insipidus in mice lacking all nitric oxide synthase isoforms. Proc Natl Acad Sci U S A. 102, 10616-21.

Mulders, S.M., Knoers, N.V., Van Lieburg, A.F., Monnens, L.A., Leumann, E., Wuhl, E., Schober, E., Rijss, J.P., Van Os, C.H., Deen, P.M., 1997. New mutations in the AQP2 gene in nephrogenic diabetes insipidus resulting in functional but misrouted water channels. J Am Soc Nephrol. 8, 242-8.

Nezic, L., Skrbic, R., Dobric, S., Stojiljkovic, M.P., Jacevic, V., Satara, S.S., Milovanovic, Z.A., Stojakovic, N., 2009. Simvastatin and indomethacin have similar anti-inflammatory activity in a rat model of acute local inflammation. Basic Clin Pharmacol Toxicol. 104, 185-91.

Nonoguchi, H., Knepper, M.A., Manganiello, V.C., 1987. Effects of atrial natriuretic factor on cyclic guanosine monophosphate and cyclic adenosine monophosphate accumulation in microdissected nephron segments from rats. J Clin Invest. 79, 500-7.

Nonoguchi, H., Sands, J.M., Knepper, M.A., 1988. Atrial natriuretic factor inhibits vasopressin-stimulated osmotic water permeability in rat inner medullary collecting duct. J Clin Invest. 82, 1383-90.

Nonoguchi, H., Sands, J.M., Knepper, M.A., 1989. ANF inhibits NaCl and fluid absorption in cortical collecting duct of rat kidney. Am J Physiol. 256, F179-86.

O'Driscoll, G., Green, D., Taylor, R.R., 1997. Simvastatin, an HMG-coenzyme A reductase inhibitor, improves endothelial function within 1 month. Circulation. 95, 1126-31.

Olsson, A.G., Lindahl, C., Holme, I., Fayyad, R., Faergeman, O., Kastelein, J.J., Tikkanen, M.J., Larsen, M.L., Pedersen, T.R., 2011. LDL cholesterol goals and cardiovascular risk during statin treatment: the IDEAL study. Eur J Cardiovasc Prev Rehabil. 18, 262-9.

Pacey, S., Gore, M., Chao, D., Banerji, U., Larkin, J., Sarker, S., Owen, K., Asad, Y., Raynaud, F., Walton, M., Judson, I., Workman, P., Eisen, T., 2010. A Phase II trial of 17-allylamino, 17-demethoxygeldanamycin (17-AAG, tanespimycin) in patients with metastatic melanoma. Invest New Drugs.

Palm, F., Teerlink, T., Hansell, P., 2009. Nitric oxide and kidney oxygenation. Curr Opin Nephrol Hypertens. 18, 68-73.

Rouch, A.J., Chen, L., Troutman, S.L., Schafer, J.A., 1991. Na+ transport in isolated rat CCD: effects of bradykinin, ANP, clonidine, and hydrochlorothiazide. Am J Physiol. 260, F86-95.

Russo, L.M., McKee, M., Brown, D., 2006. Methyl-beta-cyclodextrin induces vasopressin-independent apical accumulation of aquaporin-2 in the isolated, perfused rat kidney. Am J Physiol Renal Physiol. 291, F246-53.

Shakur, Y., Holst, L.S., Landstrom, T.R., Movsesian, M., Degerman, E., Manganiello, V., 2001. Regulation and function of the cyclic nucleotide phosphodiesterase (PDE3) gene family. Prog Nucleic Acid Res Mol Biol. 66, 241-77.

Sidaway, J.E., Davidson, R.G., McTaggart, F., Orton, T.C., Scott, R.C., Smith, G.J., Brunskill, N.J., 2004. Inhibitors of 3-hydroxy-3-methylglutaryl-CoA reductase reduce receptor-mediated endocytosis in opossum kidney cells. J Am Soc Nephrol. 15, 2258-65.

Stangherlin, A., Gesellchen, F., Zoccarato, A., Terrin, A., Fields, L.A., Berrera, M., Surdo, N.C., Craig, M.A., Smith, G., Hamilton, G., Zaccolo, M., 2011. cGMP Signals Modulate cAMP Levels in a Compartment-Specific Manner to Regulate Catecholamine-Dependent Signaling in Cardiac Myocytes. Circ Res. 108, 929-39.

Takeda, S., Kusano, E., Murayama, N., Asano, Y., Hosoda, S., Sokabe, H., Kawashima, H., 1986. Atrial natriuretic peptide elevates cGMP contents in glomeruli and in distal tubules of rat kidney. Biochem Biophys Res Commun. 136, 947-54.

Tamarappoo, B.K., Verkman, A.S., 1998. Defective aquaporin-2 trafficking in nephrogenic diabetes insipidus and correction by chemical chaperones. J Clin Invest. 101, 2257-67.

Tamma, G., Klussmann, E., Maric, K., Aktories, K., Svelto, M., Rosenthal, W., Valenti, G., 2001. Rho inhibits cAMP-induced translocation of aquaporin-2 into the apical membrane of renal cells. Am J Physiol Renal Physiol. 281, F1092-101.

Tamma, G., Klussmann, E., Procino, G., Svelto, M., Rosenthal, W., Valenti, G., 2003. cAMP-induced AQP2 translocation is associated with RhoA inhibition through RhoA phosphorylation and interaction with RhoGDI. J Cell Sci. 116, 1519-25.

Tatzelt, J., Prusiner, S.B., Welch, W.J., 1996. Chemical chaperones interfere with the formation of scrapie prion protein. EMBO J. 15, 6363-73.

Terada, Y., Moriyama, T., Martin, B.M., Knepper, M.A., Garcia-Perez, A., 1991. RT-PCR microlocalization of mRNA for guanylyl cyclase-coupled ANF receptor in rat kidney. Am J Physiol. 261, F1080-7.

Tojo, A., Gross, S.S., Zhang, L., Tisher, C.C., Schmidt, H.H., Wilcox, C.S., Madsen, K.M., 1994. Immunocytochemical localization of distinct isoforms of nitric oxide synthase in the juxtaglomerular apparatus of normal rat kidney. J Am Soc Nephrol. 4, 1438-47.

Ujiie, K., Yuen, J., Hogarth, L., Danziger, R., Star, R.A., 1994. Localization and regulation of endothelial NO synthase mRNA expression in rat kidney. Am J Physiol. 267, F296-302.

Wang, W., Li, C., Nejsum, L.N., Li, H., Kim, S.W., Kwon, T.H., Jonassen, T.E., Knepper, M.A., Thomsen, K., Frokiaer, J., Nielsen, S., 2006. Biphasic effects of ANP infusion in conscious, euvolumic rats: roles of AQP2 and ENaC trafficking. Am J Physiol Renal Physiol. 290, F530-41.

Yamada, T., Matsuda, K., Uchiyama, M., 2006. Atrial natriuretic peptide and cGMP activate sodium transport through PKA-dependent pathway in the urinary bladder of the Japanese tree frog. J Comp Physiol B. 176, 203-12.

Yang, B., Zhao, D., Verkman, A.S., 2009. Hsp90 inhibitor partially corrects nephrogenic diabetes insipidus in a conditional knock-in mouse model of aquaporin-2 mutation. FASEB J. 23, 503-12.

Yao, J.Q., Liu, Q.H., Chen, X., Yang, Q., Xu, Z.Y., Hu, F., Wang, L., Li, J.M., 2010. Hsp90 inhibitor 17-allylamino-17-demethoxygeldanamycin inhibits the proliferation of ARPE-19 cells. J Biomed Sci. 17, 30.

Zhang, S., Rahman, M., Qi, Z., Thorlacius, H., 2011. Simvastatin antagonizes CD40L secretion, CXC chemokine formation, and pulmonary infiltration of neutrophils in abdominal sepsis. J Leukoc Biol. 89, 735-42.

5

Analysis of Membrane Protein Stability in *Diabetes Insipidus*

Florian Heinke, Anne Tuukkanen and Dirk Labudde
University of Applied Sciences Mittweida
Germany

1. Introduction

Diabetes insipidus (DI) is a rare endocrine disorder, with an incidence in the general population assessed on one case per 25,000-30,000 people (Robertson, 1995; Ananthakrishnan, 2009; Krysiak, et al., 2010). It is a disease characterized by polyuria and compensatory polydipsia. The underlying causes of DI are diverse and can be central **defects**, in which no functional arginine-vasopressin is released from the pituitary, or may becaused by defects in the kidney (nephrogenic DI, NDI). Four different types of NDI are known. First, acquired NDI can originate as a side-effect of drugs, with the most prominent being the antibipolar drug lithium. Second and third, autosomal recessive and dominant inheritable NDI, are caused by gene mutations in the AQP2 gene encoding aquaporin-2. Finally, mutations in the AVPR2 gene (Deen et al., 1994; Mulders, 1998), which encodes the V2 vasopressin receptor (V2R), are the cause of the X-linked inheritable form of NDI (Fig. 1 right) (Van den Ouweland et al., 1992; Rosenthal, 1992).

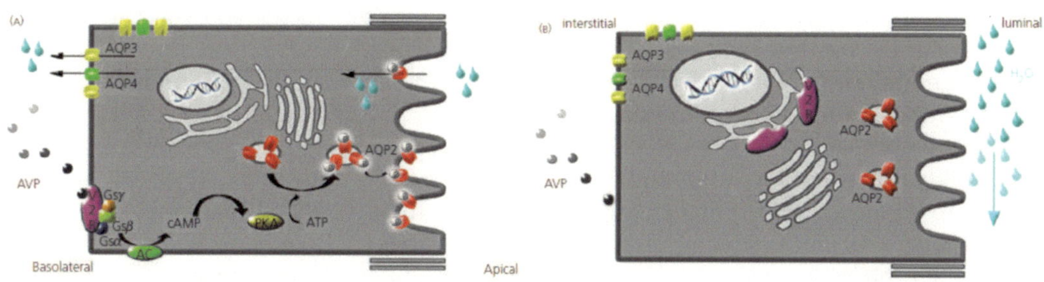

Fig. 1. Transcellular water transport in renal collecting principal duct cells and molecular cause of X-linked nephrogenic diabetes insipidus (NDI)

(Left) Vasopressin binding to its type 2 receptor (V2R) triggers a cAMP cascade that leads to the insertion of aquaporin-2 water channels in the apical membrane. This allows water to pass through this membrane and transcellular water transport to balance concentration of the pro-urine and, there by antidiuresis. (Right) In the X-linked form, NDI is often caused by V2R mutants trapped in the endoplasmic reticulum as a result of their misfolding, making them unavailable for binding arginine-vasopressin (AVP) at the basolateral plasma membrane. As a result, no transcellular water transport takes place, leading to polyuria (Los et al., 2010).

The X-linked inheritable form of nephrogenic diabetes insipidus is a disorder in which patients are unable to concentrate their urine despite the presence of the hormone arginine-vasopressin (AVP). This antidiuretic hormone regulates the process of the water reabsorption, according to the body's need, from the pro-urine that is formed by ultrafiltration in the kidney. It binds to its type 2 receptor in the kidney (Fig. 1, A). Mutations in the gene encoding the V2R often lead to NDI. Many of these mutations do not interfere with the intrinsic functionality of V2R, but cause its retention in the endoplasmic reticulum (ER) making it unavailable for AVP binding.

As a consequence of the inability of the kidneys to concentrate the pro-urine in response to AVP, diseased adult patients may have a daily output of 15–20 l of highly dilute (usually < 100 mOsmol / kg) urine. In newborn infants, NDI is characterized by irritability, poor feeding, poor weight gain and dehydration symptoms.

Classically, the diagnosis NDI was made after a dehydration test (Los et al., 2010) but it has become possible in clinical practice to apply direct analysis of the arginine vasopressin V2 receptor gene (AVPR2) and the aquaporin-2 gene for the diagnosis and differential diagnosis of nephrogenic diabetes insipidus (Fujiwara & Bichet, 2005).

To date, over 200 mutations have been described in the AVPR2 gene, which can be categorized into classes according to their cellular fate (Robben et al. 2006).

Another gene for the diagnosis of **Diabetes insipidus** is WFS1. It encodes a transmembrane protein which induces the Wolfram Syndrom (Hardy et al. 1999), a rare autosomal recessive disorder characterized by juvenile-onset non-autoimmune Diabetes mellitus, optic atrophy, sensorineural deafness and **Diabetes insipidus** (Wolfram & Wagener, 1938). In addition, psychiatric illnesses such as depression and impulsive behavior are frequently observed in affected individuals (Swift & Swift, 2001).

The minimal criteria for diagnosis are Diabetes mellitus and optic atrophy. **Diabetes insipidus**, sensorineural deafness, urinary tract anatomy, ataxia, peripheral neuropathy, mental retardation and psychiatric illness are additional symptoms seen in the majority of patients (Strom, 1998a).

The WFS1 protein, also called wolframin, consists of 890 amino acids and was predicted to have nine or ten membrane spanning domains (Inoue et al., 1998; Strom et al., 1998b). More than 100 mutations of the WFS1 gene have been identified to date in Wolfram syndrome patients. Most are inactivating mutations, suggesting loss of function to be responsible for the disease phenotype (Cryns et al., 2003). The WFS1 protein is expressed in various tissues but at higher levels in the brain, heart, lung and pancreas (Inoue et al., 1998; Strom et al., 1998b). The literature shows that the WFS1 protein is to be localized predominantly in the endoplasmic reticulum and suggested a possible role of this protein in membrane trafficking, protein processing and/or regulation of cellular calcium homeostasis (Takeda et al, 2001). A recent study showed this protein to contain nine transmembrane domains and to be embedded in the ER membrane with the amino-terminus in the cytosol and the carboxy-terminus in the ER lumen (Hofmann et al., 2003).

The short introduction shows the correlation of **Diabetes insipidus** with mutations in different membrane proteins. Membrane proteins play essential roles in cellular processes. Despite the central importance of transmembrane proteins, the number of high-resolution structures remains small due to the practical difficulties in crystalizing them. Many human disease-linked point mutations occur in transmembrane proteins. These mutations cause structural instabilities in a transmembrane protein leading it to unfold or missfold in an alternative conformation.

However, the analysis of this stability plays an important part concerning the understanding process of these diseases, especially for **Diabetes insipidus.** In this chapter, we demonstrate two different approaches on membrane protein stability analysis, results from single-molecule force spectroscopy (SMFS) on aquaporin-1 and a new method based on so called energy profiles.

2. Description of the investigated membrane proteins

The points of interest in this work are the membrane proteins: aquaporins -2, -3 and -4 as well as the arginine vasopressin V2 receptor.

2.1 Aquaporins

For a better understanding of the relationship between mutations and changes in the stability of membrane proteins, we summarize in this section the structural characteristics of water cannels. Knowledge of these aquaporins derived by experimental data revealed the affiliation of aquaporins to a family of related water channels from many species. Aquaporins provide highly permeable pores for water to cross membranes. Four identical subunits form a stable tetramer in the plane of membrane. Each subunit has a narrow pore that is selective for water passing through the middle of a bundle of α-helices. About 10 water molecules line up in a pore about 0.3 nm in diameter. Hydrophobic bonding of water with a pair of asparagine residues (Fig. 2: Asn 76 and Asn 192, human aquaporin-1 numbering) at a narrow point in the pore allows the channel to be selective for water. The monomers of the protein arose by gene duplication, since their sequences are remarkably similar. Various human tissues express 12 different aquaporin isoforms. Aquaporin-1 (Fig. 2) is found in red blood cells, retinal proximal tubules, blood vessel endothelial cells, and the choroid plexus. Aquaporin-2 is required for renal collecting ducts to reabsorb water (King et al. 2004).

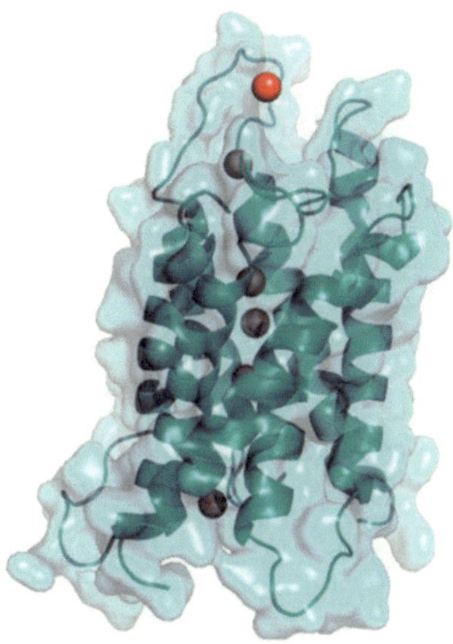

Fig. 2. Structure of an aquaprin-1 protein (PDB_ID 1ih5); The lined up water molecules are shown in red. The protein structure contains seven α-helices.

Antidiuretic hormone controls the insertion of aquaporin-2 in the collecting duct membrane. It activates a seven-helix receptor, causing cytoplasmic vesicles storing aquaporin-2 to fuse with the plasma membrane. This increases the permeability of apical plasma membranes to water, allowing it to move from the urine into the hypertonic extracellular space of the renal medulla. The water selectivity can appreciate by the protein structure. The figure 3 illustrates the network of the involved residues in the process. Additional to the exposed residue pair (Asn 76 and Asn 192) we observed Arg 195 and His 180 on the top of the pore, both closing the pore for bigger molecules or ions. The pore is hydrophobic inside. The peptide bonds of the residues Gly 188 and Ile 191 can form h-bonds with water molecules. The reaction of sensitive Cys 189 with mercuric ions closes the water pore (King et al. 2004; Pollard & Earnshaw, 2007).

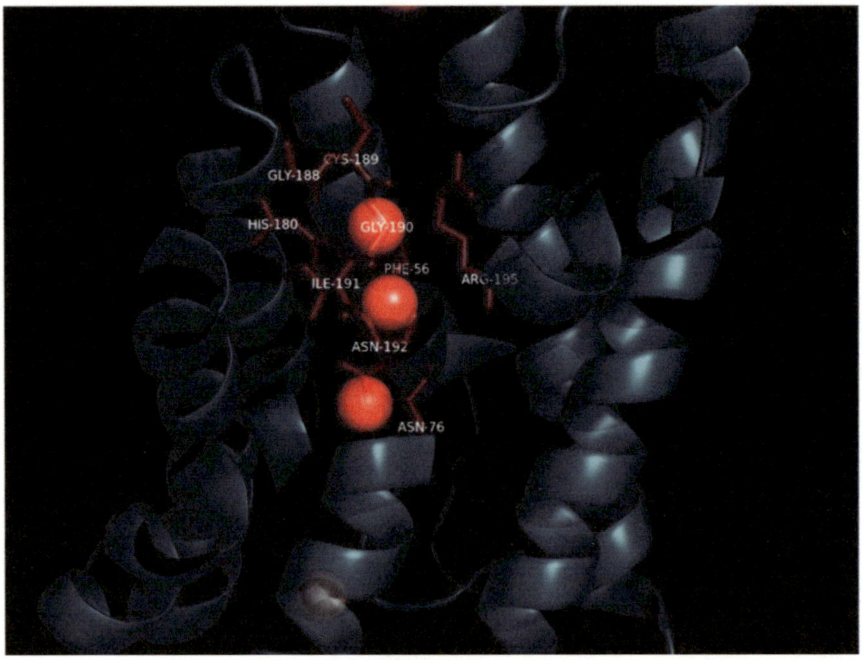

Fig. 3. Aquaporin 1 and the residue network for water transport. The following residues are involved: His 180, Gly 188, Cys 189, Gly 190, Ile 191, Asn 192, Arg 195 and Phe 56, Asn 76.

Furthermore, it is shown that two of the seven helices hold a highly conserved Asn-Pro-Ala motif (Chen et al., 2006). These two motifs meet in opposite α-helical orientation. This conformation induces a bipolar electric field changing the water molecule orientation and preventing protons to move through the channel. Further molecular simulation study has revealed a secondary free energy-barrier induced by Phe 56, His 180 and Arg 195. This barrier is located at the extracellular side, about 8 Å apart from the bipolar field. It forms a constriction region with a diameter of approximately 2 Å which allows only a single water molecule to pass the pore. Thus, the secondary free-energy barrier plays a main role in transport selectivity. Additionally, molecular dynamics simulation of Arg 195 mutants showed a significant decrease of the secondary energy-barrier leading to the loss of selectivity. This indicates that conformational changes or mutations of Arg 195 have a main influence on the transport behavior of aquaporin (de Groot et al. 2004; Chakrabarti et al., 2004a; Chakrabarti et al., 2004b; Ilan et. al, 2004).

The focus of this chapter is the analyses of the stability of membrane proteins. To collect a reliable dataset and to gather information about existing protein structures, we checked the Protein Data Bank (PDB) and the ModBase for aquaporin entries. Table 1 and table 2 give an overview over the used structures for all future calculations and discussions of the aquaporins.

Aquaporin (PDB_ID)	Sequence length (PDB)	Sequence length (Uniprot)	Number missing residues N-terminal	Number missing residues C-terminal	Coverage [%]
Aqp1/1fqy	230	273	7	36	84
Aqp4/3gd8	227	328	31	70	69
Aqp5/3d9s	251	269	1	17	93

Table 1. Overview of aquaporin structure

Aquaporin	BLAST-hit in PDB	e-Value	Model	Model-Template	reliability	Sequence identity
Aqp2:	3d9sA	2.00E-99	x	3d9sA	good	68%
Aqp3:	**1ldfA**	2.00E-46	x	3ldfA	average	43%

Table 2. Overview of models in the ModBase for the structural unknown aquaporin proteins. The highlighted (bold) PDB_ID 1ldf is the structure of a glycerol channel from *E.coli*.

While the structures of aquaporin-1, -4 and -5 have been clarified by electron crystallography (aquaporin-1) or x-ray diffraction (aquaporin-4 and -5) respectively, the structures of aquaporin-2 and -3 have been predicted by homology modeling. In homology modeling, the sequence of a structural unknown protein is queried to a protein structure database (such as the Protein Data Bank or Protein Data Bank of Transmembrane Proteins). The structure with adequate sequence identity (usually greater than 25-30%, depending on the length of the query sequence) is used as the modeling template. By simulations with force fields, using rotamer libraries and machine learning techniques, the query sequence is modeled into the given structure template and the resulting model can be evaluated. Unsuccessful modeling is caused by low sequence identity and leads to short modeled fragments or no model at all. Many of those successfully modeled structures are stored and organized in protein model databases (*e.g.* Modbase and Protein Model Portal). Because of the relatively low number of known structures finding an appropriate template is still a bottleneck in structure homology modeling.

As seen in table 2, the structure model of aquaporin-2 has been produced by using the structure of aquaporin-5 as modeling template. The most reliable structure of aquaporin-3 was modeled on the basis of a glycerol channel of *E. coli.* The neighbor joining tree (see figure 4) of aquaporin 1-5 and the glycerol channel gives insight to sequence similarity of the involved proteins and, in case of aquaporin-2 and -3 their modeling template sequences. As seen by branch length, aquaporin-2 and aquaporin-5 share the highest sequence identity in the entire tree which confirms the applicability of the aquaporin-5 structure of modeling a high reliable aquaporin-2 structure. Aquaporin-3 and the glycerol channel form a single isolated monophyletic cluster with a branch length of about 600 indicating the moderate sequence identity of 43% given in table 2. However, this sequence identity is high enough for deriving a model with an average reliability.

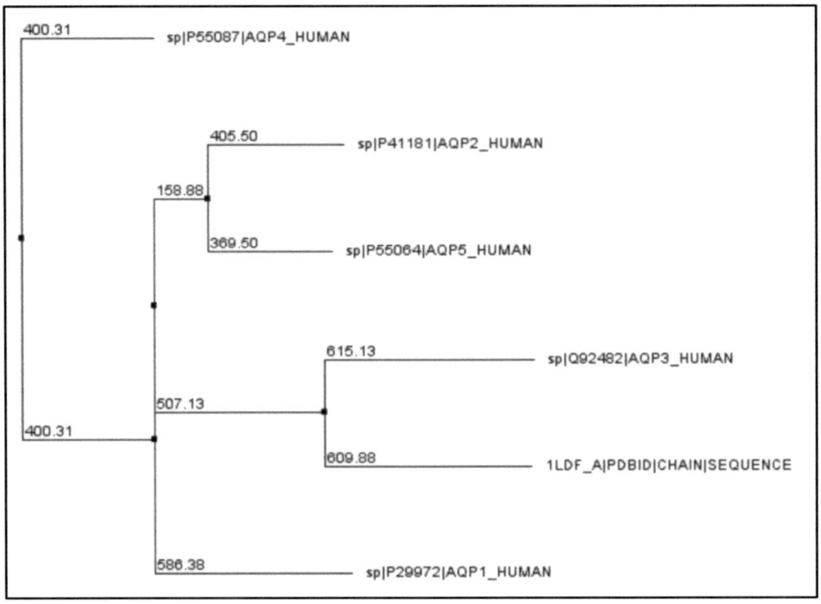

Fig. 4. The neighbor joining tree of aquaporin 1-5 and the glycerol channel of *E. coli* (PDB_ID 1ldf) indicates the sequence similarities of aquaporin-2,-3 and their modeling templates aquaporin-5 and 1ldf, respectively. The direct neighborhood of the involved proteins and their template structures point to the adequate reliability of the existing aquaporin-2 and aquaporin-3 models.

Mutations in aquaporin are correlated with NDI. For the detailed analyses of mutations in aquaporin-2, we concentrated on two well-defined point mutations. Characterization of D150E and G196D aquaporin-2 mutations are responsible for nephrogenic diabetes insipidus: importance of a mild phenotype. These two mutations were compared with the wild-type protein (aquaporin-2-wt) for functional activity (water flux analysis), protein maturation, and plasma membrane targeting. As shown by Guyon et al (2009) the D150E mutant induces an intermediate water flux compared to the aquaporin-2 –wt whereas the G196D mutant leads to no water flux. This observation is consistent with results from immunocytochemical experiments and Western blotting which indicate partial targeting of D105E in plasma membrane and complete sequestration of G196D within intracellular compartments. When coinjecting aquaporin-2-wt with mutants, no (aquaporin-2-wt + D150E) or partial (aquaporin-2-wt + G196D) reduction of water flux were observed compared with aquaporin-2-wt alone, whereas complete loss of function was found when both mutants were coinjected (Guyon, et al., 2009).

2.2 Model of V2 receptor

The V2 receptor belongs to the class A of G-protein-coupled receptors containing seven membrane spanning helices which are connected by extracellular and intracellular loops of varying length. The function of V2R is coupled to the G-protein activating adenyl cyclase (Barberis et al. 1998). If an agonist arginine vasopressin binds to V2R, the receptor becomes activated which leads to allosteric structural rearrangements. These structural changes then enable interactions with the cytosolic G-protein. The binding site of arginine vasopressin on the V2 receptor is formed within the transmembrane helices II –VII (Slusarz et al. 2006). Regions between residues 88-96, 119-127, 284-291 and 311-317 contain most of the residues involved in binding. The selectivity of vasopressin was proposed to be connected with non-conserved residue Q180 whose carboxamide forms hydrogen bonds with carboxamide of Asn5 in the peptide. The stability of the hormone in the bound state is ensured by two hydrogen bonds between peptide backbone atoms of Tyr 2 and Asn 5. In general, hydrogen bonding and salt bridges were identified as the most important interactions contribution to the arginine vasopressin binding (Slusarz et al. 2006). Significant hydrophobic interactions were not detected.

A three-dimensional structural model of human V2 receptor (Fig. 5) was produced using I-TASSER protein structure modeling pipeline (Roy et al. 2010). I-TASSER builds protein models using multiple threading alignments on template structures and iterative assembly. The top three structural templates used in the structure prediction were PDB_ID 2ks9 (Substance-P receptor) with sequence identity of 19 %, PDB_ID 2rh1 (B2-adrenergic G protein-coupled receptor) with sequence identity of 22 % and PDB_ID 1l9h (bovine rhodopsin) with sequence identity of 18 % to VR2 receptor. The modeled structure was subjected first to conjugate gradient minimization and then MD simulation using the program NAMD2 (Phillips et al. 2005) and the CHARMM27 force-field (MacKerrel et al. 1998). The TIP3P solvent model represented the water molecules (Joergensen et al. 1983). Simulations assumed constant particle number, constant pressure and constant temperature (*NpT*) ensembles. *Langevin* dynamics was used to maintain constant temperature and pressure was controlled using a hybrid *Nose-Hoover Langevin* piston method. Extensive molecular dynamics simulations were done on the modeled structure in order to study its quality and structural stability. The average root-mean-square-deviation of the backbone atoms of the modeled structure during the simulation was found to be 2.7 Å. The model structure has seven helical segments: helix I 34 -64, helix II 73 - 101, helix III 109 - 142, helix IV 153-175, helix V 202-230, helix VI 248-296, helix VII 304-328.

Molecular dynamics (MD) simulation is one of the most common methods to study computationally protein function, conformational flexibility, and interactions. It is a technique to calculate the equilibrium and transport properties of a classical many-body system (Frenkel, 2002). In MD simulations, particles obey the laws of classical mechanics and the technique show how the system of particles evolves in time. The first MD simulation of a protein was done in the 1970s in vacuum for duration of 10ps (McCammon et al. 1977). Nowadays, the computational power allows simulation of about one million atoms, up to 100 Å in size and time scale up to 1 microsecond. Even single membrane proteins in the native lipid environment can be studied. Simulations of large biomolecular systems are becoming more feasible as demonstrated by the work on the MD-based structure prediction of the ribosome complex from *E. coli* (Villa, 2009), the simulation of the assembly of lipids and proteins into lipoprotein particles (Shih, 2007), the MD studies of viral capsid self-assembly (Freddolino, 2006; Miao, 2010) and vesicle fusion simulations (Kasson, 2010). MD simulations are used to gain information about the conformational changes of protein structure, *i.e.* sample the configuration space. In addition, MD simulations provide thermal averages of molecular properties such as the free energy change upon binding or atomic mean square fluctuation amplitudes. According to the ergodic hypothesis all microstates of a system are equally probable for a particle over a long period of time. Hence, the average of a process parameter over time and the average over the statistical ensemble are the equal. Simulation can be used to study the dynamics of a system in detail by observing the conformational states that are accessible in a given temperature. *Ab initio* structure prediction starting from amino acid sequence of a protein using MD simulations is computationally feasible only for very small proteins, but simulations can be used to improve computational predicted protein structures obtained by homology modeling or fold recognition. The limitations of MD simulations are still relatively short time scale, inaccuracies in the description of physical interactions and the size limitation of the simulation system.

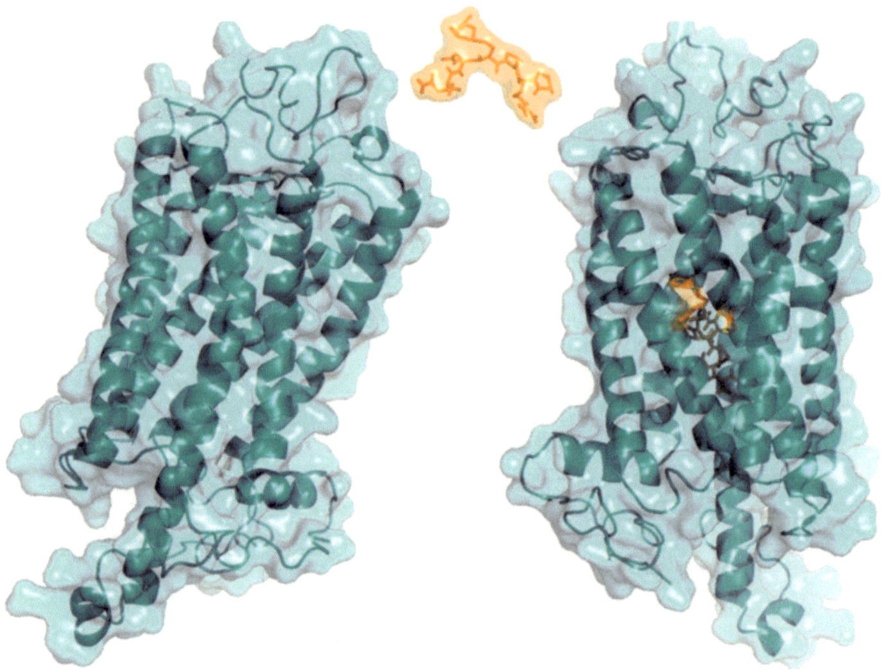

Fig. 5. Structure model of the V2 receptor (left). On the right side a result from Molecular Docking Server. The AVP hormone is highlighted in orange and is bound to the V2 receptor (right).

Mutation	Effect
A84D	This mutation not only affects receptor folding in such a way as to lead to its retention inside the intracellular compartments but, as expected, also has profound effects on its binding and coupling properties (pubmed_Id 10820167).
I130F	Functional analysis of I46K and I130F revealed reduced maximum agonist-induced cAMP responses as a result of an improper cell surface targeting (pubmed_Id 10770218,16006591)
P322S	P322S mutation of AVPR2 gene leads to a mild form of CNDI. (pubmed_Id 10026830,9402087)

Table 3. Overview of mutations in the V2 receptor and a short description of the biological effect. (More mutants in the appendix.)

In this work we address only a repertory. We do not analyses mutations cause constitutive activation of the receptor in this work (such as: Feldman et al, 2005). The table 3 shows the position and the molecular description of the investigated mutations of the V2 receptor be focused on this work.

3. SMFS – Stability and experiments

Atomic force microscopy (AFM) is mostly known for its imaging capabilities (Müller & Engel, 1999; Müller, et al, 1999; Seelert et.al, 2003). Recently, single-molecule force spectroscopy (SMFS) has proven to be a tool for detecting and locating inter- and intra-molecular forces on a single molecule level. SMFS experiments allow measuring the stability of membrane proteins and also probing the energy landscapes (Janshoff et al., 2000; Janovjak et al, 2004). In Fig. 6A a schematic representation of the force spectroscopy instrumentation is shown. Molecules with complex three-dimensional structures, such as proteins, can be unfolded in a controlled way. When transmembrane proteins are unfolded in force spectroscopy experiments, during continuous stretching of the molecule the applied force is

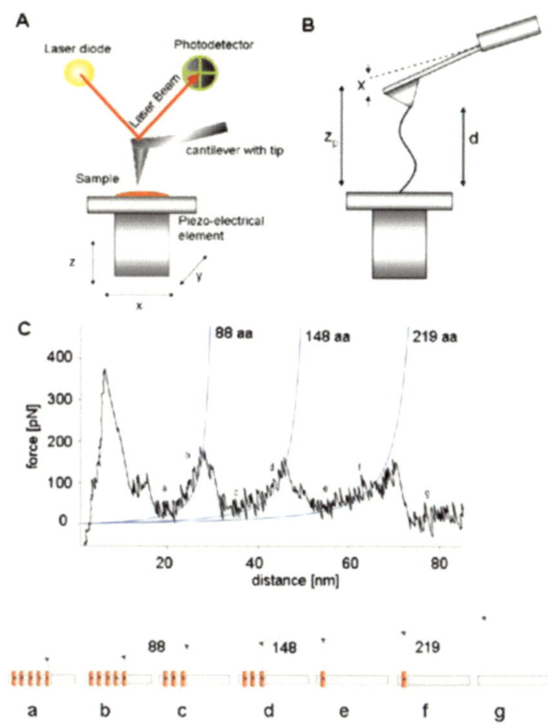

Fig. 6. A: Schematic representation of AFM. The sample is mounted on a piezo-electric element and scanned under a sharp tip attached to the cantilever. The voltage difference of the photodetector is proportional to the deflection of the cantilever.
B: Unfolding of a transmembrane protein. A single molecule is attached between the tip and the sample while the distance between tip and sample is continuously increased.
C: Typical spectrum obtained from an unfolding experiment of bR with the main peaks fitted by a hyperbolic function (WLC model) and correlated to the unfolding of secondary structure elements (cartoon at the bottom).

measured by the deflection of the cantilever and plotted against extension (tip-sample separation), yielding a characteristic force-distance curve (F-D curve) (see Fig. 6). From the analysis of single molecule force spectra it is possible to associate the peaks to individual stable structural segments within membrane proteins. For a given protein under study, the F-D curves exhibit certain patterns, which contain information about the strength and location of molecular forces established within the molecule, stable intermediates and reaction pathways, and the probability with which they occur. For membrane proteins the sequence of the unfolding peaks follow the amino acid sequence of the protein. Fitting each peak to a hyperbolic function, the worm-like chain model (WLC), gives the number of already unfolded amino acids (Rief et al. 1997).
Consequently, with the peaks and the predicted secondary structure, it is possible to associate the peaks to structural domains (see Fig. 7 and Fig. 8). Force curves show specific and unspecific interactions which lead to different unfolding pathways.
To draw biologically relevant conclusions on molecular interactions about how strong they are and where they occur, or whether they are independent or occur only in presence with other events, one must analyze many F-D curves by identical objective procedures. Thus, there is an increasing demand for data analysis techniques that offer fully automated processing of many datasets with identical analysis procedures. To discriminate force spectra showing specific and non-specific interactions and different unfolding/unbinding pathways, classification and pattern recognition algorithms are urgently needed (Marcico et al. 2007; Sapra et al., 2008).
One aim of the analyses of experimental data from SMFS measurements is the detection of possible unfolding pathways. Furthermore, we can identify different groups in hierarchical trees, which relate to different unfolding events. These events correspond to secondary structure elements and stabilized regions in the investigated protein.

3.1 SMFS experiments on aquaporin-1

Here, we work on data from SMFS experiments for human aquaporin-1 from the literature In the work of (Möller et al, 2003) 26 F-D curves were measured and manually aligned. The individual hAQP1 molecules were unfolded by pulling at their C-termini. The author created an overlay of all investigated curves (Fig. 7).

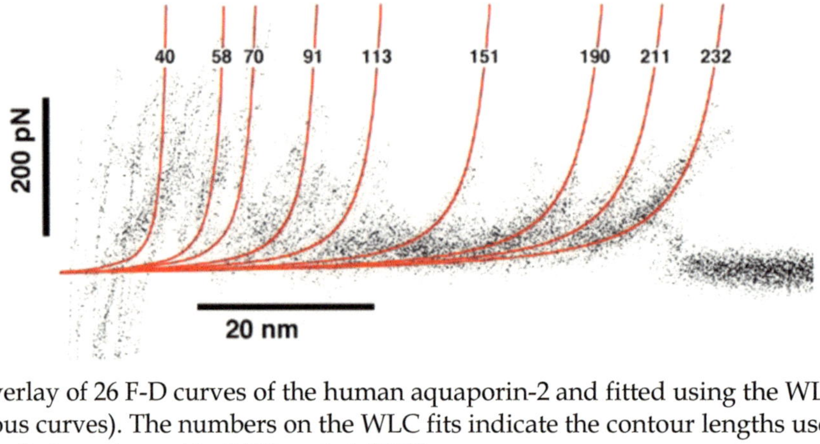

Fig. 7. Overlay of 26 F-D curves of the human aquaporin-2 and fitted using the WLC model (continuous curves). The numbers on the WLC fits indicate the contour lengths used to obtain the fit, in amino acids (Möller et al, 2003).

The next step is the mapping of the unfolding results of the known structure of aquaporin-1. This leads to a correlation of unfolding events and the secondary structure of the membrane protein. A possible description of all events is listed in table 4.

Contour length from WLC fits (aa)	Peak occurrence number/percent (n_{total} = 26)	Average force (pN)	Proposed potential barrier	Grey marker (Fig. 8)
40 ± 8	26 (100%)	206 ± 64	end of helix H6	1
58 ± 6	24 (92%)	157 ± 49	end of helix HE	2
70 ± 8	17 (65%)	125 ± 63	end of helix H5	3
91 ± 7	22 (85%)	156 ± 44	Helix H5	4
113 ± 7	13 (50%)	98 ± 54	end of helix H4	5
151 ± 5	20 (77%)	82 ± 53	Helix H3	6
190 ± 10	17 (65%)	98 ± 33	end of helix HB	7
211 ± 6	16 (62%)	77 ± 42	HelixH2	8
232 ± 5	26 (100%)	152 ± 62	HelixH1	9

Table 4. Contour lengths, peak occurrence, average forces, and positions of potential barriers in Aqp1 topology by SMFS experiments (additional link to Fig. 8 – topology).

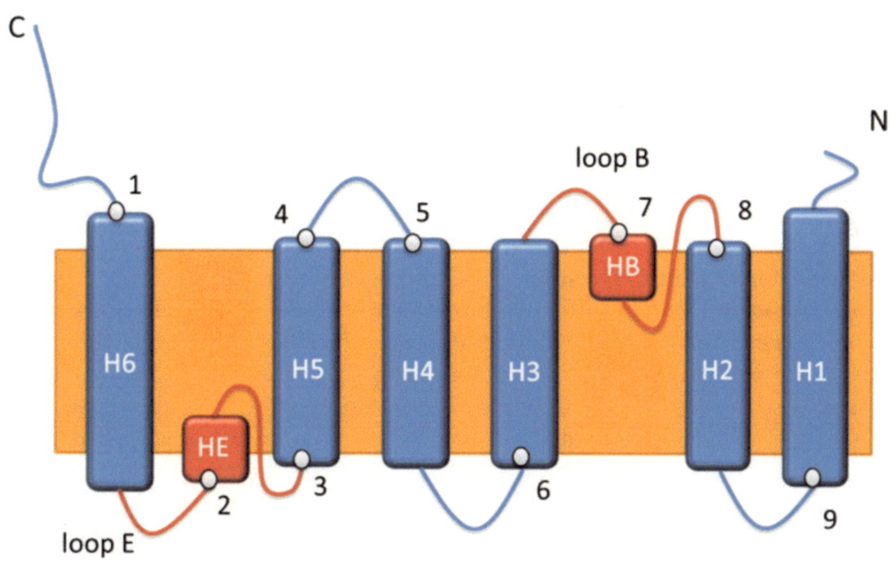

Fig. 8. Topology model of Aqp1: Shown are the secondary structure elements in the lipid bilayer, as described by the 3D structure. Numbers in ovals represent the numbers of proposed potential barrier of table 4.

Interesting are the two long loops, with formed helices in the transmembrane region. A view of the structure of aquaporin-1 quickly shows the role of both helices (HB and HE). The residues Asn 72 (part of HB) and Asn 192 (part of HE) arrange the immediate place of the pore (Fig. 8 and 9).

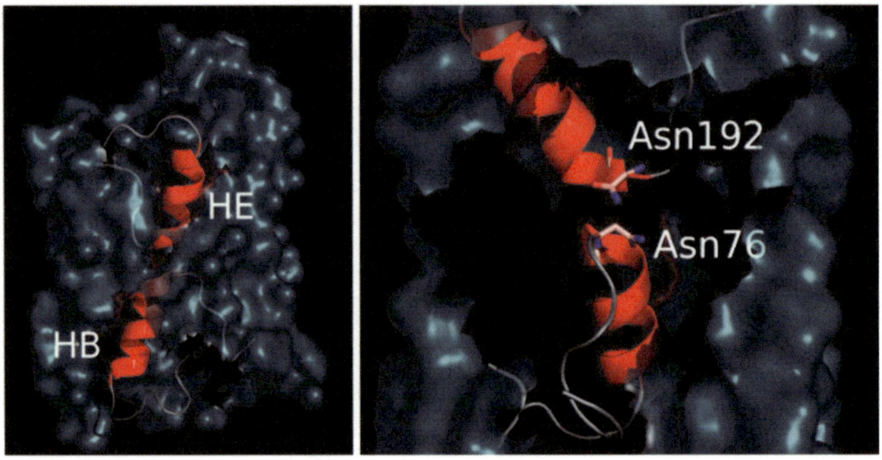

Fig. 9. Structure of aquaporin-1: Left side loop regions E and B (transmembrane helices HE and HB highlighted in red), right: Interface with conserved residues Asn 192 and Asn 76.

This important functional and structural feature corresponds to two unfolding events in aquaporin-1. The major force peak appeared within the noisy region but at a tip-membrane separation of about 20 nm. The WLC fit (Fig. 7 red line - 58 aa) showed an average contour length of 58±6 amino acids, while the rupture event exhibited an average force of 147±49 pN. According to the topology shown in Fig. 8, the extracellular end of helix HE is separated from the C-terminal end. Thus, this adhesion peak is likely to reflect the unfolding of HB. We can observe an analog situation for the loop B and the corresponding helix HB.
The force peaks found at a contour length of 190±10 amino acids (Fig.7) exhibit an average rupture force of 98±33 pN. This distance from the C-terminus corresponds to helix HB, which dips into the membrane from the cytoplasmic side and is only 11 amino acids long. Thus, this adhesion peak is likely to reflect the unfolding of HB.

3.2 Unfolding characteristic of aquaporin-2 and aquaporin-3

On the basis of known structures of aquaporin-1,-4 and -5 and the models of the aquaporin-2 and -3 we created a multiple structure alignment using the PDBeFold service of the EMBL-EBI. We clustered the resulting q-scores of all pair wise structural alignments by applying the UPGMA method (Unweighted Pair Group Method with Arithmetic Mean) to get a rooted tree (see Fig. 10, left). The inner node of the tree indicates that the known structures of aquaporin-5 and the glycerol channel (PDB_ID 1ldf) are almost identical in protein fold. The direct neighborhood of the aquaporin-1 structure and the models of aquaporin-2 and -3 give a strong hint for the unfolding characteristics of aquaporin-2. Due to their high structural similarity we postulate that aquaporin-2,-3 have a similar unfolding characteristic in comparison to aquaporin-1. The pair wise structural alignment of aquaporin-2 and -3 is shown in Fig. 10, right. The structure of aquaporin-4 shares a high similarity to the other structures.

4. Energy profiles – Stability and theory

A lot of tools and methods in the field of bioinformatics and structural biology are based on structure and/or sequence comparison. In this section we demonstrate a new method based on so called energy profiles for analyzing protein structure stability. Those profiles are

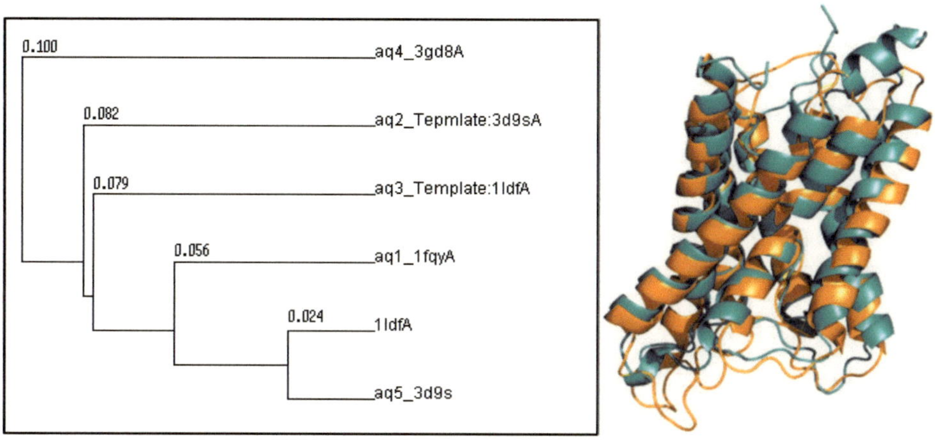

Fig. 10. Left: tree of the q-scores resulting from the PDBeFold service using Unweighted Pair Group Method with Arithmetic Mean (UPGMA) hierarchical clustering. Right: A structural alignment of aquaporin-1 structure (orange) and the model of aquaporin-2 (cyan).

calculated by coarse grained models. Based on the residue contacts in known protein structures, we calculated the potential for pair wise residue-residue-interactions. An energy profile is a schematic plot of the interaction energy of each residue as a function of the residue position in the sequence.

4.1 Theory of energy profiles

In this section, we show the theoretical aspects and calculation of so called protein energy profiles. The aspects explained in this section are essential in understanding the energy profile based methods we applied to the aquaporin proteins.

Energy profiles are derived by coarse-grained amino acid interaction models based on information of known protein structures. In general, the energy of any protein is given by equation (1), where e^*_{ij} acts as the interaction energy between two amino acids a_i and a_j. The function $f(r_{ij})$ quantifies e^*_{ij} by the Euclidean distance r_{ij}. The solvent interaction energy of an amino acid a_i is given by e'_{i0} and is relativized by expression $g(i)$, which describes the solvent accessibility state of a_i.

$$E = \sum_{<ij>} e_{ij} f(r_{ij}) + \sum_{i} e'_{i0} g(i) \qquad (1)$$

Based on (1), we designed a coarse grained interaction scheme, which uses the C_α and C_β coordinates of the amino acids. Furthermore we redefined $g(i)$ and $f(r_{ij})$. Instead of using a continuous space, $f(r_{ij})$ acts as Boolean function. That means, depending on r_{ij}, amino acid a_i is either interacting with amino acid a_j or it is not. Based on the work of (Dressel et al. 2007; Wertz & Scheraga, 1978) we defined a cut-off threshold for r_{ij} of 8Å. That leads to the equation (2).

$$f(r_{ij}) = \begin{cases} 1 & \text{if } r_{ij} \text{ is} \leq 8\text{Å}, \\ 0 & \text{else.} \end{cases} \qquad (2)$$

ÅFurthermore we introduced an amino acid specific inside/outside-property which reflects the orientation of the amino acid side chains with respect to the center of mass of the neighboring residues and was defined in the following way:
A residue is declared as inside, if

$$\left|\vec{C}_{\alpha}-\vec{c}\right|<5 \vee\left(\vec{C}_{\alpha}-\vec{C}_{\beta}\right)\left(\vec{C}_{\alpha}-\vec{c}\right)<0 \tag{3}$$

$\vec{C}_{\alpha/\beta}$ are the vectors of the $C_{\alpha/\beta}$ atoms, $\vec{c}$ is the center of mass of all amino acids in a surrounding sphere with a radius of 5Å. For determining the center of mass only C_{α} atoms are taken into account. Using this property the inverse Boltzmann equation can be applied to calculate the energy of each amino acid a_i in the protein structure by (4).

$$e_i=-k_B T \ln\left(\frac{n_{(i,in)}}{n_{(i,out)}}\right) \tag{4}$$

The parameters $n_{(i,in)}$ and $n_{(i,out)}$ are equal to the number of inside and outside occurrences of amino acid a_i, respectively. These parameters are derived by known globular and membrane protein structures. In our coarse grained model, the interaction energy e_{ij} between two amino acids a_i and a_j is equal to the summation of e_i and e_j. Finally, let S be a set of amino acids, let $k = |S|$ and a_i is defined as the observed amino acid. For each $a_j \in S$ is $r_{ij} \leq 8$Å. Then the total energy E_i of a_i equals (5). By iterating over all amino acids in a protein structure the total energy for each amino acid can be calculated and the energy profile is generated.

$$E_i=\sum_{j=1}^{k}\left(e_i+e_j\right)=\sum_{i=1}^{k}\left(-k_B T \ln\left(\frac{n_{(i,in)}}{n_{(i,out)}}\right)-k_B T \ln\left(\frac{n_{(j,in)}}{n_{(j,out)}}\right)\right) \tag{5}$$

Additionally, it needs to be said that we discard further solvent interaction calculation (seen in the second summation in equation 1) because these information is modeled by the amino acid specific inside/outside-property. In addition, we declared T as constant which leads to discarding the constant $-k_B T$ in the energy profile calculation. Thus the energies, which result by our model, are arbitrary unit entities [a.u.] and are direct proportional to energies given in [J] or [kcal·mol^{-1}].
In conclusion, by calculating the total energy of an amino acid in a protein structure, physicochemical and structural information are abstracted to one single value.
The relation of amino acid stability and amino acid energy is explainable by the folding of the protein and its energy landscape. As one of the last steps in protein biosynthesis the polypeptide folds into the native protein structure state spontaneously which is equal to the proteins most stable fold. This process can be described as a function of the loss of the Helmholtz free energy within an amino acid interaction energy state. Commonly a folded protein in its stable state holds the minimized amount of free energy. The energy profile is a transformation of the energy landscape of the protein at the point of minimized free energy, which leads to the conclusion that the energy value of an amino acid a_i given by an energy profile is a transformation of the stability of the amino acid a_i in the structure. Figure 11 illustrates the resulting energy profile (right) of the structure model of aquaporin-2 (left).

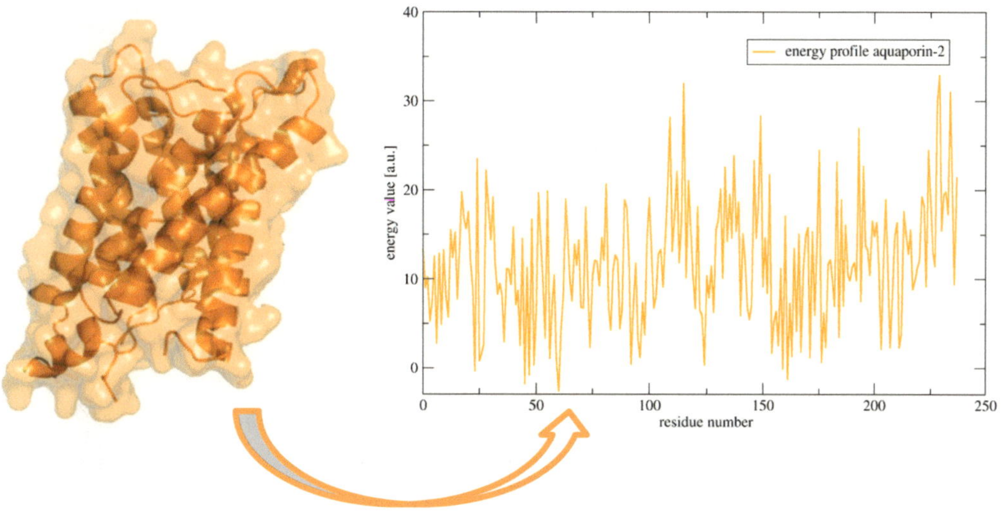

Fig. 11. Left: Structure model of aquaporin-2 and the corresponding energy profile (right) of this model.

4.2 Energy profiles analyses of the investigated aquaporins

On the basis of the so-called energy profiles we can compare the structures and models of all investigated aquaporins, well-defined mutations and the influences of mutations for the stability of the aquaporins.

4.2.1 Energy profiles of the investigated aquaporins

For calculating the energy profiles we used the structures given in table 1 and table 2. To evaluate the energy profiles we checked the already existing aquaporin models concerning their reliability. As shown, the best matching structures were used as template structures for homology modeling. On the level of energy profiles we can confirm our hypothesis that all investigated aquaporins have the same stability characteristics. For this purpose we created a multiple energy profile alignment (MEPAL). We adapted standard algorithms in clustering and deriving consensus profiles and energy conservation. Figure 12 shows the MEPAL for all of the involved aquaporins in **Diabetes Insipidus** and the human aquaporin-1.

The MEPAL method is based on classical multiple sequence alignment algorithms using modified scoring functions optimized for energy profile comparison. The tree (see Fig. 13) is calculated by applying the UPGMA clustering method to the pair wise distance scores which are calculated by the MEPAL algorithm. Furthermore, the graphical alignment output (Figure 12) consists of three parts. The upper row shows the energetically aligned energy profiles represented by the amino acids of the protein sequence which are colored depending on their energy. The greater the energy of an amino acid the greater is the red color content. The middle row shows the consensus profile. In the consensus profile, each energy at position *i* is derived by calculating the pair wise distance sores of all aligned energies at position *i*. The energy with the lowest average distance is representing the consensus profile at position *i*. Finally, the bottom row shows the conservations at each alignment position. Each conservation value is calculated by the sum of pair wise energy distances and is normalized by the number of aligned profiles (Gusfield 1993, Gusfield 1997).

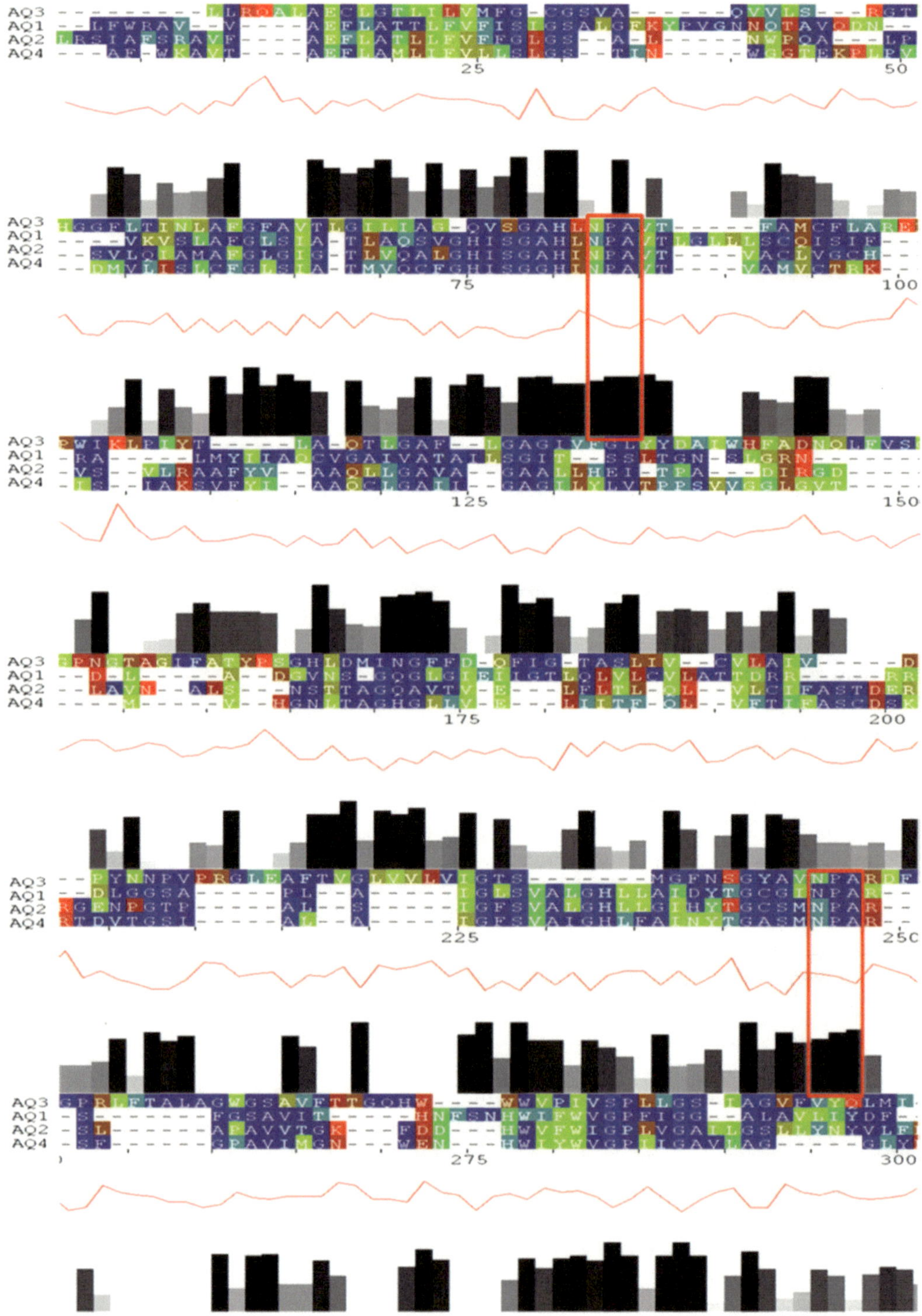

Fig. 12. MEPAL output for the energy profile alignment of aquaporin-1, -2,- 3 and -4. The Asn-Pro-Ala motifs are highlighted by red boxes.

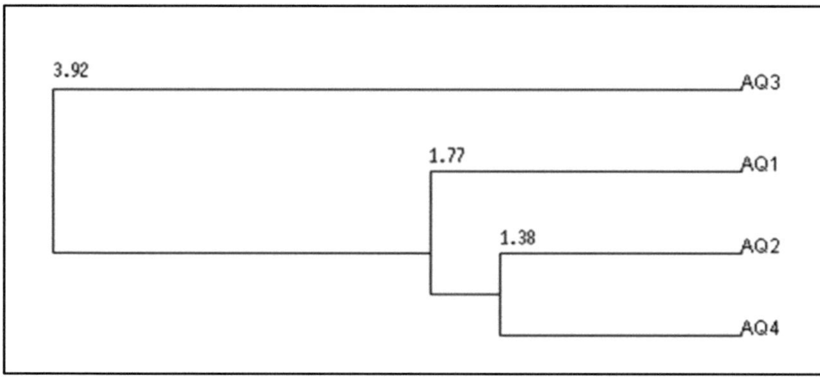

Fig. 13. UPGMA tree, based on energy profiles of aquaporin-1, -2, -3 and -4.

The energy profile alignment based UPGMA Tree, which was calculated by MEPAL indicates high similarities between the energy profiles of aquaporin-1,-2 and -4 and is seen in figure 13. The distance of 3.92 between aquaporin-3 and the other structures corresponds to significant similarity. The graphical output of the MEPAL illustrates several highly energetically conserved amino acids and regions. Two of these conserved regions correspond to the opposite orientated Asn-Pro-Ala motifs in helix HB and helix HE (see section 2.1). These two motifs are highlighted by red boxes in Fig. 12. The energetic conservation of these motifs and their surrounding amino acids confirms the importance of these residues in water transport in aquaporin. Additionally the residues Gly 188, Phe 56, Cys 189, Ile 191 and His 180, which are involved in water transport as well, show differences in sequential and energetic conservation. In detail the conserved amino acids Gly 188 and Phe 56 show slight divergences or no divergences at all concerning their calculated energy. Cys 189 and Ile 191 show no conservation in aquaporin 1-4; but these changes have no effect on the level of energy profiles. Missing in aquaporin-3, His 180 shows sequential and energetic conservation in the other aquaporins. We postulate that these slight divergences do not affect the water flux significantly.

A further point of interest lies in Arg 195. This residue is conserved in all four proteins but varies energetically. These divergences arise from conformational changes of the residue and the structural environment. Based on the facts we referred to in section 2.1, we postulate that these divergences between aquaporin 1-4 lead to a change in the secondary free-energy barrier influencing the transport selectivity and the water flux. It also needs to be said that the significant differences in the energy profile progression between aquaporin-3 and the other structures (see Fig. 13) might result by the less reliable aquaporin-3 model. Despite these divergences, we can confirm our postulated similarities concerning the unfolding characteristics of the aquaporins involved in **Diabetes Insipidus**.

4.2.2 Energy profiles and stability of the mutants of aquaporin-2

For comparison on the level of energy profiles we generated aquaporin-2 models with the two mutations: D150E and G196D. Based on all three models we calculated the energy profiles and created a MEPAL. The results lead to a distance tree and can be discussed on the level of aligned energy profiles (Fig.14).

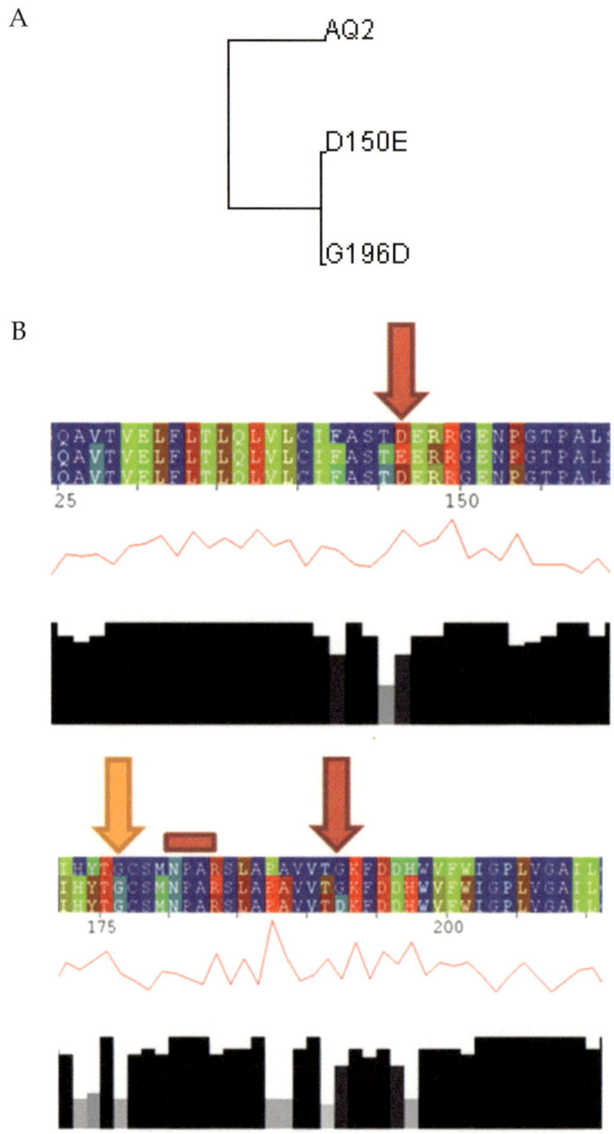

A: The UPGMA tree of the resulting distance scores of the energy profiles calculated by MEPAL. The inner node indicates that these point mutations lead similar energy profiles.
B: The MEPAL output of the investigated energy profiles. The point mutations induce various energetic changes which are highlighted by arrows. The red rectangle illustrates the Asn-Pro-Ala motif.

Fig. 14. Results from the analyses of the energy profile of aquaporin-2 and the investigated mutants.

The energy profile based UPGMA tree (see Fig. 14, A) indicates strong similarities between the energy profiles of the two modelled aquaporin-2 mutants. This leads to the conclusion that both mutants induce the same energetic, structural and functional changes. While both mutations led to energetic variations in the entire energy profiles we focused our discussion on the mutations sites (see Fig. 14, B - red arrows). It needs to be said that because of the modelling procedure and the energy profile calculation the resulting energy profile covers not all amino acids of the mutated sequence. In this case, this leads to an index indention of 3 amino acids. The mutation D150E (see Fig. 14, B - at the top) induces an energetically increase of the two surrounding residues decreasing the energetic conservation at these positions. Interestingly, in this region the mutation G196D induces almost the same energetic increase as D150E. At the mutation site of the modelled G196D variant (see Fig. 14, B - at the bottom), the mutation induces slight energetic divergences in the region where the mutation site is located. Furthermore, in this region the G196D mutation leads to the same energetic variations as the D150E mutation. This observation can be confirmed at nearly all positions in the energy profiles of the modelled aquaporin mutations. Interestingly, both mutations do not affect the energetic conservation of the Asn-Pro-Ala motif (highlighted by a red rectangle in Fig. 14, B at the bottom).

Additionally, we point to the energetic changes of Gly 188 (highlighted by an orange arrow in 14 B at the bottom). As mentioned in section 2.1 this residue is involved in water transport. Both mutations lead to an energetically increase of Gly 188 and reduce the energetic conservation in these three investigated energy profiles. Thus, we postulate that the mutations D150E and G196D affect the transecullar water transport.

4.3 Energy profiles analyses of the V2 receptor

For investigating energetic influences, binding capabilities and the effect of mutations in the V2 receptor we generated a V2 receptor model by molecular modeling. This model was used to calculate the energy profile of this receptor. Furthermore, we used the Molecular Docking Server to process a docking simulation of the V2 receptor model and the arginine vasopressin hormone. The structure of the model and its hormone in docked state was used for further analyses. Both models are illustrated in Fig. 5 in subsection 2.2. We calculated the energy profile of the V2 receptor model in docked state to detect energetic divergences induced by conformational changes and the hormone itself. Thus, AVP is an oligopeptide it can be integrated into the energy profile calculation in the way it is explained in section 4.1.

To detect docking induced energetic changes both derived energy profiles were aligned using the MEPAL method. The alignment revealed energetic divergences in the surrounding of the amino acids Ala 84 (Fig. 15, A), Ile 130 (Fig. 15, B) and Pro 322 (Fig. 15, C). This leads to the conclusion that these amino acids are involved in hormone binding. Mutations of these amino acids are well described in literature and are causing a loss in functionality and hormone affinity (see table 3). Our novel energy profile based approach brought more evidence to these described mutations.

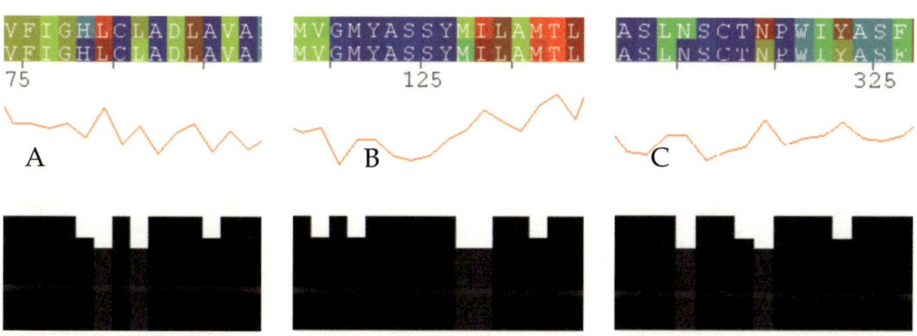

Fig. 15. MEPAL output for the energy profile alignment of fragments of V2 receptor and the complex

5. Discussion of the stability of the investigated membrane proteins

The antidiuretic hormone, ADH, also called vasopressin and arginine-vasopressin, is a nanopeptide (nine amino acids) synthesized in the hypothalamus, transported to and stored in the posterior lobe of the pituitary gland which releases it into the blood circulation. It has antidiuretic and vasopressor actions. The effects of vasopressin result from stimulation of V1 and V2 receptors, V1 mainly responsible for vasoconstriction, V2 for the antidiuretic effect V1 receptors are coupled by G-protein to phospholipase C. V2 receptors are coupled by G-protein to adenylcyclase. Its activation elicits an increase in cAMP which, via protein kinases, induces the activation of aqueous channel aquaporin-2 -mainly located in the renal collecting duct. Under the influence of vasopressin aquaporin-2 migrates from the cytoplasm to the apical membrane. In **nephrogenic diabetes insipidus** there are aquaporin-2 alterations.

Aquaporin-3 is constitutively expressed in the basolateral membrane of the cell. When water floods into the cell through aquaporin-2 channels, it can rapidly exit the cell through the aquaporin-3, 4 channels and flow into blood.

We investigated the stability of membrane proteins on the basis of experimental and theoretical assumptions. Membrane proteins play essential roles in cellular processes. These mutations cause structural instabilities in a transmembrane protein leading it to unfold or missfold in an alternative conformation. By the structural comparison of the aquaporin-1, investigated by SMFS, with the involved proteins and protein models, we can postulate that aquaporin-2,-3 and -4 exhibit similarities in unfolding characteristics. This assumption can be confirmed by our theoretical approach. These theoretical methods are based on the so called energy profile calculation which is explained in this work. On the basis of stability analyses and the application of energy profile based methods we were able to enforce evidence for water flux reduction induced by well described mutations. Furthermore the correlation of residue conservation and energetic conservation of amino acids involved in water transport was detected. Especially the role of the two conserved helices HB and HE could be detected and described on the basis of experimental and theoretical methods.

For analyzing the V2 receptor we derived a structure model by molecular modeling and processed AVP docking simulations. As a main part we focused on selected point mutations and their influences in hormone affinity. Thus, we were able to enforce evidence described in literature.

6. Acknowledgment

This project was funded by the Free State of Saxony and the University of Applied Sciences Mittweida. The authors thank Daniel Stockmann for helpful discussions, motivations and powerful programming.

7. Appendix

In the preparation of the book chapter we collected the literature for well-defined mutations in the V2 receptor. We don't claim to have a complete list or all description. On the basis of this list we compared our results in the context of the docking model of the complex V2 receptor and the AVP hormone.

Mutation	Effect
N22Q	N-linked glycosylation at asparagine 22, Mutagenesis of asparagine 22 to glutamine abolished N-linked glycosylation of the V2 receptor (N22Q-V2R), without altering its function or level of expression. (pubmed_Id 10362843)
L44F	the mutant L44F and the in vitro mutant S167A were expressed in their mature form at wild-type levels (pubmed_Id 8863826)
L44P	mutants L44P, W164S, S167L, and S167T lacked complex glycosylation and were expressed at low levels, mutants misfolded (pubmed_Id 8863826,16006591)
S45C	Strong beta-catenin (CTNNB1) expression in the tumor cells and identified a heterozygote missense Ser45Cys mutation of exon 3 of CTNNB1 (pubmed_Id 19294427).
I46K	Functional analysis of I46K and I130F revealed reduced maximum agonist-induced cAMP responses as a result of an improper cell surface targeting (pubmed_Id 10770218)
L62P	core-glycosylated mutants L62P and V226E were excluded from lysosomes (pubmed_Id 18048502)
A84D	this mutation not only affects receptor folding in such a way as to lead to its retention inside the intracellular compartments but, as expected, also has profound effects on its binding and coupling properties (pubmed_Id 10820167).
A98P	the cell-surface expressions of mutant receptors were totally (A98P and L274P) (pubmed_Id 17371330)
W99R	Mutation of a tryptophan located at the beginning of the first extracellular loop (W99R) that greatly impaired the binding properties of the receptor and had a minor effect on its intracellular routing (pubmed_Id 10820167).
F105V	the F105V mutation is delivered to the cell surface and displayed an unchanged maximum cAMP response, but impaired ligand binding abilities of F105V were reflected in a shifted concentration-response curve toward higher vasopressin concentrations. As the extracellularly located F105 is highly conserved among the vasopressin/oxytocin receptor family, functional analysis of this residue implicates an important role in high affinity agonist binding. (pubmed_Id 10770218)
R113W	The cell-surface expressions of mutant receptors were totally (A98P and L274P) or partially (R113W) absent. V2R-R113W, -G201D, and -T204N were expressed in the ER and in the basolateral membrane as immature, high-mannose glycosylated, and mature complex-glycosylated proteins. The immature forms of V2R-R113W and -T204N, but not V2R-G201D, were rapidly degraded. The mature forms varied extensively in their stability and were degraded by only lysosomes (V2R-T204N and wild-type V2R) or lysosomes and proteasomes (V2R-G201D, -R113W). (pubmed_Id 17371330,16006591,7984150,10770218)

I130F	Functional analysis of I46K and I130F revealed reduced maximum agonist-induced cAMP responses as a result of an improper cell surface targeting (pubmed_Id 10770218,16006591)
R137C	(R137C) in the second intracellular loop, which has been associated with constitutive activation of the AVPR2. In conclusion, adults with intermittent, severe hyponatraemia may have a constitutively activating mutation in the AVPR2 with resultant nephrogenic syndrome of inappropriate antidiuresis. R137C gain-of-function mutation was detected by means of mutation analysis of the V2R gene. (pubmed_Id 18753429,18622631,16843086,19179480,17229917)
R137L	V2R-R137L mutant interacts with beta-arrestins in an agonist-independent manner resulting in dynamin-dependent internalization. V2R-R137L mutant traffic considerably more efficiently to the plasma membrane than V2R-R137H, identifying this as a potentially important mutation-dependent difference affecting V2R function. (pubmed_Id 19179480,16843086)
R143P	R143P and delta V278 mutants are retained within the cytoplasmic compartment. (pubmed_Id 7560098)
S167A	The mutant S167A was functionally active, (pubmed_Id 8863826)
R181C G185C	loss of receptor function (pubmed_Id 15841479)
G201D	the complex-glycosylated mutant G201D were partially located in lysosomes, G201D was expressed in the ER and in the basolateral membrane as immature, high-mannose glycosylated, and mature complex-glycosylated proteins. (pubmed_Id 18048502,16006591)
R202C	R202C mutant reaches the cell surface, a simple binding impairment at the cell surface (pubmed_Id 7560098)
T204N	degraded by only lysosomes, T204N was expressed in the ER and in the basolateral membrane as immature, high-mannose glycosylated, and mature complex-glycosylated protein (pubmed_Id 16006591)
Y205C Y205F Y205H	-for Y205C the lack of a Tyr residue at position 205 is responsible for the abolished receptor function rather than the formation of a disastrous second disulfide bond. Y205C mutant was almost inactive. -Analysis of the intermolecular interaction of the Tyr-205 hydrogen group by molecular modeling showed that Tyr-205 was located in transmembrane domain (TM) 5, and that its hydroxy group formed a hydrogen bond with Leu-169 main-chain =O located in TM 4. The mutation of Tyr-205 to phenylalanine would cause loss of this hydrogen bond and decrease or change the interaction between these TM coils, thus affecting the ability of AVP to bind to the receptor. According to this molecular model of AVPR2, the Y205F mutation would cause nephrogenic diabetes insipidus. - the loss of receptor function of Y205H, NDI-causing mutation Y205H which affects a codon frequently found to be mutated to Cys in NDI patients. (pubmed_Id 15841479,11026555, 17216256,)
V206D	stimulation of the V206D mutant increased the cAMP accumulation only slightly, V206D was mainly expressed in the endoplasmic reticulum (ER) as immature proteins. (pubmed_Id 11026555,16006591)

F287L	F287L mutant in COS-7 cells revealed significant dysfunction and accumulate intracellular cyclic adenosine monophosphate in response to AVP hormone stimulation. (pubmed_Id 11916004)
P322S	P322S mutation of AVPR2 gene leads to a mild form of CNDI. (pubmed_Id 10026830,9402087)
S363A	The S363A mutation that confers recycling to the V2R did not alter its interaction with arrestins. (pubmed_Id 11353798)

Table appendix: Overview of mutations in the V2 receptor and a short description of functional and structural influences.

8. References

Robertson GL (1995) Diabetes insipidus. *Endocrinol Metab Clin North Am* 24: 549-572.

Ananthakrishnan S (2009) Diabetes insipidus in pregnancy: etiology, evaluation, and management *Endocr Pract* 15: 377-382.

Krysiak, R.; Kobielusz-Gembala, I. et al (2010) Recurrent pregnancy-induced diabetes insipidus in a woman with hemochromatosis Endocrine Journal, online-ISSN: 1348-4540

Deen PM, Verdijk MA, Knoers NV, Wieringa B, Monnens LA, van Os CH, van Oost BA.Requirement of human renal water channel aquaporin-2 for vasopressin-dependent concentration of urine. *Science* 1994; 264: 92–95.

Mulders SM, Bichet DG, Rijss JPL, Kamsteeg EJ, Arthus MF, Lonergan M, Fujiwara M,

Morgan K, Leijendekker R, van der Sluijs P, van Os CH, Deen PMT. An aquaporin-2 water channel mutant which causes autosomal dominant nephrogenic diabetes insipidus is retained in the Golgi complex. *J Clin Invest* 1998; 102: 57–66.

Van den Ouweland AMW, Dreesen JCFM, Verdijk M, Knoers NVAM, Monnens LAH, Rocchi M, VanOost BA. Mutations in the vasopressin type-2 receptor gene (Avpr2) associated with nephrogenic diabetes-insipidus. *Nat Genet* 1992; 2: 99–102.

Rosenthal W, Seibold A, Antaramian A, Lonergan M, Arthus MF, Hendy GN, Birnbaumer M, Bichet DG. Molecular-identification of the gene responsible for congenital nephrogenic diabetes-insipidus. *Nature* 1992; 359: 233–235

Los, E. L .; Deen, P. M. T; Robben, J. H. Potential of Nonpeptide (Ant)agonists to Rescue Vasopressin V2 Receptor Mutants for the Treatment of X-linked Nephrogenic Diabetes Insipidus. *Journal of Neuroendocrinology* 2010; 22: 393–399

Fujiwara TM, Bichet DG. Molecular biology of hereditary diabetes insipidus. J AmSoc Nephrol. 2005;16:2836–46.

Robben JH, Knoers NVAM, Deen PMT. Cell biological aspects of the vasopressin type-2 receptor and aquaporin 2 water channel in nephrogenic diabetes insipidus. Am J Physiol Renal Physiol 2006; 291: F257–F270.

Hardy, C.; Khanim, F.; Torres, R. et al. Clinical and Molecular Genetic Analysis of 19 Wolfram Syndrome Kindreds Demonstrating a Wide Spectrum of Mutations in WFS1. Am. *J. Hum. Genet.* 1999; 65:1279–1290.

Wolfram, D.J. and Wagener, H.P. (1938) Diabetes mellitus and simple optic atrophy among siblings: report on four cases. *Mayo Clinic Proc.*,13, 715–718.

Swift, M. and Swift, R.G. (2001) Psychiatric disorders and mutations at the Wolfram syndrome locus. *Biol. Psychiatry*, 47, 787–793.

Strom, T.; Hörtnagel, K.; Hofmann, S. Diabetes insipidus, diabetes mellitus, optic atrophy and deafness (DIDMOAD) caused by mutations in a novel gene (wolframin) coding for a predicted transmembrane protein. *Human Molecular Genetics*, 1998, Vol. 7, No. 13: 2021–2028

Inoue, H., Tanizawa, Y., Wasson, J., Behn, P., Kalidas, K., Bernal-Mizrachi, E., Mueckler, M.,

Marshall, H., Donis-Keller, H., Crock, P. et al. (1998) A gene encoding a transmembrane protein is mutated in patients with diabetes mellitus and optic atrophy (Wolfram syndrome). *Nat. Genet.*, 20, 143–148.

Strom, T.M., Hoetnagael, K., Hofmann, S., Gekeler, F., Scharfe, C., Rabl, W., Gerbitz, K.D. and Meitinger, T. (1998) Diabetes insipidus, diabetes mellitus, optic atrophy and deafness (DIDMOAD) caused by mutations in a novel gene (wilframin) coding for a predicted transmembrane protein. *Hum. Mol. Genet.*, 7, 2021–2028.

Cryns, K., Sivakumaran, T.A., Van den Ouweland, J.M., Pennings, R.J., Cremers, C.W., Flothmann, K., Young, T.L., Smith, R.J., Lesperance, M.M. and Van Camp, G. (2003)

Mutational spectrum of the WFS1 gene in Wolfram syndrome, nonsyndromic hearing impairment, diabetes mellitus, and psychiatric disease. *Hum. Mut.*, 22, 275–287.

Takeda, K., Inoue, H., Tanizawa, Y., Matsuzaki, Y., Oba, J., Watanabe, Y., Shinoda, K. and Oka, Y. (2001) WFS1 (Wolfram syndrome 1) gene product: predominant subcellular localization to endoplasmic reticulum in cultured cells and neuronal expression in rat brain. *Hum. Mol. Genet.*, 10, 477–484.

Hofmann, S., Philbrook, C., Gerbitz, K.D. and Bauer, M.F. (2003) Wolfram syndrome: structural and functional analyses of mutant and wild-type wolframin, the WFS1 gene product. *Hum. Mol. Genet.*, 12, 2003–2012.

King LS, Kozono D, Agre P. From structure to disease: the evolving tale ofaquaporin biology. *Nat Rev Mol Cell Biol.* 2004 5(9):687-98. Review.

Pollard TD, Earnshaw, WC. (2007), *Cell Biology*, Springer, ISBN 978-3-8274-1861-6, Heidelberg

Guyon C, Lussier Y, Bissonnette P, Leduc-Nadeau A, Lonergan M, Arthus MF, Perez RB, Tiulpakov A, Lapointe JY, Bichet DG. Characterization of D150E and G196D aquaporin-2 mutations responsible for nephrogenic diabetes insipidus: importance of a mild phenotype. *Am J Physiol Renal Physiol.* 2009;297(2):F489-98.

Ambrish Roy, Alper Kucukural and Yang Zhang, TASSER: a unified platform for automated protein structure and function prediction. *Nat Protoc.* 2010 April; 5(4): 725–738

D. Frenkel and B.J. Smit. Understanding Molecular Simulation. From Algorithms to Applications. Elsevier, 2002.

Jr. A. D. MacKerell, D. Bashford, M. Bellott, R. L. Dunbrack Jr., J. D. Evanseck, M. J. Field, S. Fischer, J. Gao, H. Guo, S. Ha, D. Joseph McCarthy, L. Kuchnir, K. Kuczera, F. T. K. Lau, C. Mattos, S. Michnick, T. Ngo, D. T. Nguyen, and B. Prodhom. All-atom empirical potential for molecular modeling and dynamics studies of proteins. *J. Phys. Chem. B*, 1998.

J. A. McCammon and M. Karplus. Internal motions of antibody molecules. *Nature*, 268(5622):765{766, Aug 1977.

Peter L. Freddolino, Anton S. Arkhipov, Steven B. Larson, Alexander McPherson, and Klaus Schulten. Molecular dynamics simulations of the complete satellite tobacco mosaic virus.*Structure*, 14:437-449, 2006.

Assembly of lipids and proteins into lipoprotein particles. Amy Y. Shih, Anton Arkhipov, Peter L. Freddolino, Stephen G. Sligar, and Klaus Schulten. Assembly of lipids and proteins into lipoprotein particles *Journal of Physical Chemistry B*, 111:11095-11104, 2007.

Yinglong Miao, Peter J. Ortoleva, Viral structural transition mechanisms revealed by multiscale molecular dynamics/order parameter extrapolation simulation. *Biopolymers* Volume 93, Issue 1, pages 61–73, January 2010Peter M. Kasson, Erik Lindahl, and Vijay S. Pande. Atomic-resolution simulations predict a transition state for *vesicle* fusion defined by contact of a few lipid. *PLoS Computational Biology, 2010* June; 6(6): e1000829.

Jorgensen, W. L.; Chandrasekhar, J.; Madura, J. D.; Impey, R. W.; Klein, M. L. Comparison of simple potential functions for simulating liquid water. *J. Chem. Phys* 1983, *79*, 926-935.

James C. Phillips, Rosemary Braun Wei Wang James Gumbart, Emad Tajkhorshid, Elizabeth Villa, Christophe Chipot, Robert D. Skeel, Laxmikant Kalé, Klaus Schulten, Scalable molecular dynamics with NAMD

Barberis C, Mouillac B, Durroux T.,*J Endocrinol.* 1998 6(2):223-9. Structural bases of vasopressin/oxytocin receptor function.

Slusarz MJ, Giełdoń A, Slusarz R, Ciarkowski J. Analysis of interactions responsible for vasopressin binding to human neurohypophyseal hormone receptors-molecular dynamics study of the activated receptor-vasopressin-G(alpha) systems. *J Pept Sci.* 2006 Mar;12(3):180-9.

Feldman BJ, Rosenthal SM, Vargas GA, Fenwick RG, Huang EA, Matsuda-Abedini M, Lustig RH, Mathias RS, Portale AA, Miller WL, Gitelman SE.: Nephrogenic syndrome of inappropriate antidiuresis., N Engl J Med. 2005 352(18):1884-90.

Müller, D.J., Engel, A.: Voltage and pH-induced channel closure of porin OmpF visualized by atomic force microscopy. J. Mol. Biol. 285, 1347–1351 (1999)

Müller, D.J., Sass, H.J., Muller, S.A., Buldt, G., Engel, A.: Surface structures of native bacteriorhodopsin depend on the molecular packing arrangement in the membrane. *J. Mol.Biol.* 285, 1903–1909 (1999)

Seelert, H., Dencher, N.A., Muller, D.J.: Fourteen protomers compose the oligomer III of the proton-rotor in spinach chloroplast ATP synthase. *J. Mol. Biol.* 333, 337–344 (2003)

Janshoff, A., Neitzert, M., Oberdorfer, Y., Fuchs, H.: Force spectroscopy of molecular systems-single molecule spectroscopy of polymers and biomolecules. *Angew Chem. Int. Ed.* Engl. 39(18), 3212–3237 (2000)

Janovjak, H., Struckmeier, J., Hubain, M., Kedrov, A., Kessler, M., Muller, D.J.: Probing the energy landscape of the membrane protein bR. *Structure* 12(5), 871–879 (2004)

Rief, M., Gautel, M., Oesterhelt, F., Fernandez, J.M., Gaub, H.E.: Reversible unfolding of individual titin immunoglobulin domains by afm. *Science* 276(5315), 1109–1112 (1997)

Marsico A, Labudde D, Sapra T, Muller DJ, Schroeder M. A novel pattern recognition algorithm to classify membrane protein unfolding pathways with high-throughput single-molecule force spectroscopy. *Bioinformatics.* 2007

Sapra KT, Balasubramanian GP, Labudde D, Bowie JU, Muller DJ. Point mutations in membrane proteins reshape energy landscape and populate different unfolding pathways. *J Mol Biol.* 2008 Feb 29;376(4):1076-90.

Möller C, Fotiadis D, Suda K, Engel A, Kessler M, Müller DJ. Determining molecular forces that stabilize human aquaporin-1. *J Struct Biol.* 2003 Jun;142(3):369-78.

Chen H, Wu Y, Voth GA. Origins of proton transport behavior from selectivity domain mutations of the aquaporin-1 channel., *Biophys J.* 2006;90(10):L73-5.

de Groot, B. L., T. Frigato, V. Helms, and H. Grubmüller. 2003. The mechanism of proton exclusion in the aquaporin-1 water channel. *J. Mol. Biol.* 333:279–293.

Chakrabarti, N., E. Tajkhorshid, B. Roux, and R. Pomes. 2004. Molecular basis of proton blockage in aquaporins. *Structure.* 12:65–74.

Chakrabarti, N., B. Roux, and R. Pome`s. 2004. Structural determinants of proton blockage in aquaporins. *J. Mol. Biol.* 343:493–510.

Ilan, B., E. Tajkhorshid, K. Schulten, and G. A. Voth. 2004. The mechanism of proton exclusion in aquaporin channel. *Proteins.* 55: 223–228.

Dressel, F., Tuukkanen, A., Schroeder M., and Labudde, D., Understanding of SMFS barriers by means of energy profiles, *Proc. GCB*, 2007

Wertz, D. H. and Scheraga, H. A., Influence of water on protein structure. An Analysis of the preferences of amino acid residues for the inside or outside and for specific conformations in a protein molecule. *Macromolecules.* 1978 Jan-Feb;11(1):9-15.

Gusfield D., Efficient Methods for Multiple Sequence Alignment with Guaranteed Error Bounds, *Bulletin of Mathematical Biology*, Vol. 55, p. 141-154, 1993

Gusfield D., Algorithms on Strings, Trees and Sequences, Cambridge University Press, 1997

6

New Insights into the Diagnosis and Management of Pregnancy-Related Diabetes Insipidus

Carmen Emanuela Georgescu
Department of Endocrinology,
"Iuliu Haţieganu" University of Medicine and Pharmacy Cluj-Napoca
Romania

1. Introduction

Diabetes insipidus in pregnancy (*diabetes insipidus gravidarum*, gestational diabetes insipidus or pregnancy-related diabetes insipidus) is considered to be a rare disease complicating up to 1 in 25000-30000 pregnancies; however, emerging evidence suggests that often the disease is under-diagnosed (Aleksandrov et al., 2010). As stated by the Italian E. Momigliano, in 1929, in his first monograph on 31 cases of pregnancy-related diabetes insipidus (Momigliano, 1929), the disease may occur in an apparently healthy woman, during any stage of pregnancy, usually in the latter half, or may aggravate during pregnancy when previously diagnosed. As a paradox, the disorder may disappear days to weeks after delivery, or may alleviate, or remain unaltered (Bleakley, 1938). Moreover, aggravated recurrence of the disorder in successive pregnancies is recognized (Blotner & Kunkel, 1942).

Interest towards pregnancy-related diabetes insipidus revived about 20-30 years ago, once it became apparent that this clinical condition is closely associated with liver disease, HELLP syndrome and the wide spectrum of preeclampsia, all with potentially serious consequences on the maternal course of gestation and fetal health and development.

The aim of the present book chapter is to review the body water homeostasis during pregnancy as well as to insist on clinical conditions associated with the occurrence of diabetes insipidus in pregnancy and the early postpartum period. Not only true gestational diabetes insipidus will be addressed but, notably, maternal hypothalamic-pituitary diseases associated with diabetes insipidus presenting high incidence during pregnancy and the postpartum period will be detailed. It is the author's hope that at the end of the chapter, the reader will find answers to hot questions on the intimate mechanisms facilitating gestational diabetes insipidus, the need to screen or not for alterations in water metabolism in pregnant women at risk, the challenges in differential diagnosis of arginin-vasopressin (AVP) disturbances in a pregnant women and the associated clinical conditions including preeclampsia, acute fatty liver and HELLP (*Hemolysis-Elevated Liver enzymes-Low Platelets*) syndrome.

In addition, etiological considerations on AVP deficiency or defective hormone action in the fetus and neonate will be made.

2. General adaptations of the endocrine system and the maternal hypothalamic-pituitary axis to pregnancy

The fetal-placental unit develops as a unique endocrine organ in pregnancy to account for various endocrine changes. It synthesizes large amounts of hormones; in turn, these synthesis products are secreted into the fetal and maternal circulation. After 8 weeks of gestation, the placenta is the main source of progesterone, which derives from maternal LDL-cholesterol. Most of placental progesterone enters the maternal circulation and hence maternal progesterone plasma concentrations gradually raise during pregnancy up to 150 ng/ml. Likewise, 17ß-estradiol and estrone are produced by the placenta *via* conversion from both maternal and fetal DHEA-S, whereas estriol is formed in the placenta from fetal adrenal DHEA-S as the primary source. In both mother and child, serum human chorionic gonadotropin (hCG) levels increase progressively to reach a peak at 10-14 weeks of pregnancy and thereafter fall until delivery. Undoubtedly, hCG is involved in steroidogenesis and maintenance of the corpus luteum activity during the first weeks of gestation. Unlike hCG, the plasma levels of human placental lactogen hormone (hPL) increase throughout the pregnancy to plateau at term. Human PL is secreted mostly into maternal circulation to induce lipolysis, resulting in increased availability of free fatty acids; it inhibits glucose uptake and gluconeogenesis in the mother, all these metabolic effects predisposing to maternal insulin resistance and hyperinsulinemia. Recently, human placental growth hormone (hPGH) synthesis was certified in pregnant women; it gradually replaces pituitary GH during pregnancy and is supposed to promote placental and fetal growth (Chellakooty et al., 2002).

In order to adapt to fetal requirements, pregnancy *per se* is associated with considerable changes in the maternal endocrine status, including physiological changes of the osmoregulatory system. Some of the most significant changes occur in the anterior pituitary and thyroid glands to meet the nutritional needs of the fetus. The pituitary gland enlarges during normal gestation due to estrogen- and to a lesser extent progesterone-induced hyperplasia of lactotroph cells, explaining 10-fold increased maternal prolactin (PRL) levels by the end of pregnancy. By the 6th to 7th week of pregnancy, basal and stimulated GH release from the maternal pituitary is suppressed *via* placental GH-induced IGF-1 synthesis (Chellakooty et al., 2002). By the same time, follicle-stimulating (FSH) and luteinizing hormone (LH) levels start to decrease along to their response to gonadotropin-releasing hormone (GnRH) stimulation.

Iodine requirements are increased in the pregnant woman up to 200-300 μg daily due to accelerated renal clearance and transplacental passage of inorganic iodine to supply fetal needs. Additional mechanisms consist of increased thyroid hormones demands to compensate for high thyroxin binding globulin (TBG) levels in the mother, stimulation of the thyroid gland by the thyrotropin-like activity of hCG, and activity of the type 3 placental deiodinase (Glinoer, 1997).

The hypothalamic-pituitary-adrenal axis is subjected to significant changes during pregnancy as evidenced by increased maternal cortisol levels, mainly because of an increase in the concentration of corticosteroid binding globulin (CBG), and reduced cortisol clearance. But it is also observed that free cortisol levels are higher during the second trimester and plateau in the third. Several mechanisms are thought to be involved: an altered set point for ACTH, effects of placental ACTH on adrenal hormone production, antiglucocorticoid actions of progesterone, and cortisol resistance (Karaca et al., 2010).

Notably, the placental 11ß-hydroxysteroiddehydrogenase efficiently protects the fetus from maternal hypercortisolism by cortisol inactivation. In addition, placental synthesis of CRH is demonstrated. Placental CRH is under the control of cortisol by positive feed-forward and behaves as a determinant of onset of parturition (Kalantaridou et al., 2003).
Both estrogen and progesterone activate synthesis of renin and, subsequently, production of angiotensin II and aldosterone, respectively. Nevertheless, the maternal vasculature becomes refractory to the pressor effects of angiotensin II, a phenomenon essential to blood volume expansion during pregnancy. Moreover, the physiological action of aldosterone is counteracted by progesterone, a competitive inhibitor of aldosterone in the distal tubule.

3. Water balance, arginin-vasopressin metabolism, aquaporin-2 expression and vasopressinase activity in pregnancy

3.1 Hemodynamic changes and water metabolism in normal pregnancy

Pregnancy is a physiological condition associated with water retention which is especially prominent in the last trimester. Studies of body fluid volume regulation in normal human pregnancy pointed out towards water retention leading subsequently to increased total blood volume and decreased plasma osmolality. In both humans and rats, a 30–50% increase in extracellular fluid, plasma and blood volume was reported (Schrier & Briner, 1991). At 6 weeks of pregnancy, an early decrease in systemic and renal vascular resistance with under-filling of the arterial system is documented. As compensatory mechanisms, this will induce sympathetic system stimulation and enhanced cardiac output as well as activation of the renin-angiotensin-aldosterone (RAA) system with associated renal sodium and water retention, leading to the abovementioned expansion of total plasma volume. Evidence of arterial vasodilatation as a primary event of the hyper-dynamic circulatory status in pregnancy is offered by animal studies, such as the rat. Indeed, this appears to be a hormone-triggered mechanism, since up-regulation of endothelial nitric oxide synthase (eNOS) by estradiol has been documented. In line with this finding, increased expression of the eNOS gene in the aorta wall, and elevated plasma nitrite and nitrate levels were detected in pregnant rats. Moreover, neural NOS expression was also found to be increased in the hypothalamus of pregnant rats. In turn, inhibition of the NOS activity has been shown to result in a reverse of renal and systemic vascular changes and normalization of cardiac output (Schrier & Ohara, 2010).
Pregnancy-mediated vasodilatation itself results in non-osmotic AVP release from the hypothalamus. During pregnancy, the osmotic threshold at which pregnant women manifest thirst and release AVP is shifted to a level lower to that of non-pregnant women (Lindheimer & Davison, 1995). Subsequently, a decrease of about 10 mOsm/kg in plasma osmolality ensues starting with the 6th week of pregnancy. Similar changes may be induced in non-pregnant women in whom exogenous hCG is administered (Davison et al., 1988).
Thus, reduction in arterial pressure of more than 10-20% releases AVP from the posterior pituitary by lowering the osmoregulatory system set point, an effect mediated by stimulation of baroreceptors located in the walls of the left atrium and large arteries and leading *via* the glossopharyngeal and vagal nerve to the CNS and then the hypothalamus. Nevertheless, non-osmotic AVP release is not unique during physiological pregnancy but also occurs in adrenal insufficiency, pathological low-output congestive cardiac failure or liver cirrhosis, in the last triggered by splanchnic arterial vasodilatation. Likewise, orally active non-peptide-selective V_2 receptor antagonists administered to patients with cardiac

failure or cirrhosis of the liver increase urinary water excretion while reversing hyponatremia (Schrier et al., 1998). Eventually, the non-osmotic AVP stimulation during pregnancy will promote water retention and increased body fluid volume with plasma hypoosmolality. Figure 1 presents hemodynamic changes and adaptations of water and AVP metabolism during normal pregnancy.

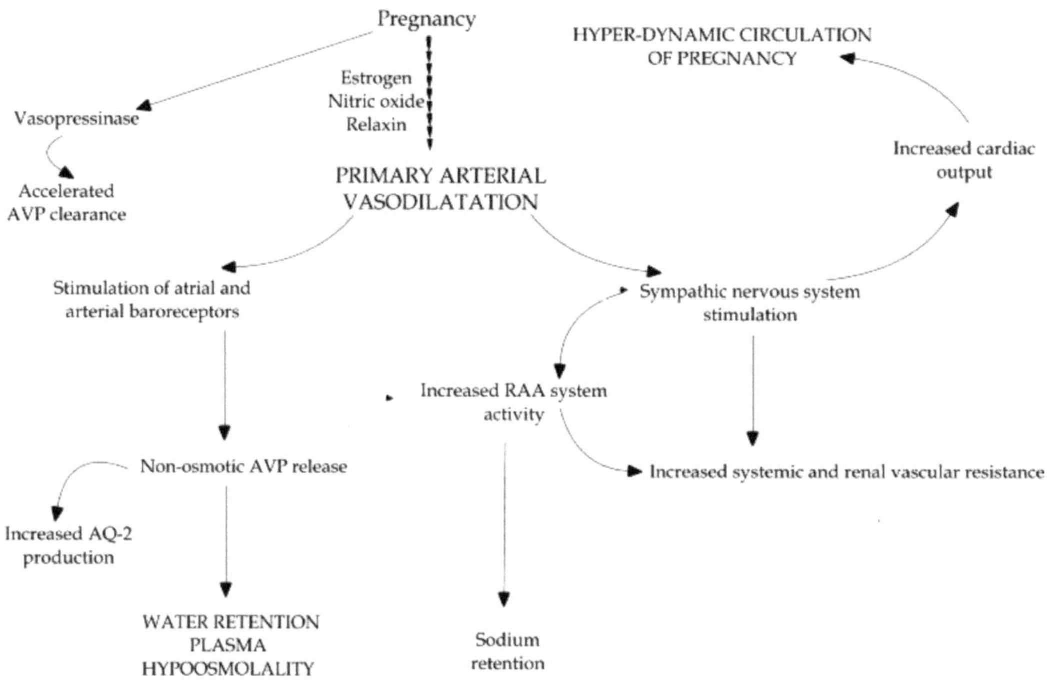

Fig. 1. Hemodynamic changes and adaptations of water and AVP metabolism in normal pregnancy.

3.2 Aquaporin-2 and vasopressinase activity in normal pregnancy

Water molecules transport across membranes is mediated by water channel proteins called aquaporins. Of the several isoforms of aquaporins identified in the kidney and other organs (brain, liver, pancreas, colon, spleen, lung, submandibular gland, testes, leukocytes), aquaporin-2 is abundant in the collecting duct principal cells and is the main target for AVP effects to mediate water transport across the apical membrane of the renal collecting duct. In response to AVP, aquaporin-2 is translocated from cytoplasmic vesicles to apical plasma membranes by shuttle trafficking to increase water permeability of the membrane. After ending AVP stimulation, aquaporin-2 is redistributed and stored into cytoplasmic vesicles.

Excretion of aquaporin-2 in the urine can be quantified and it appears that urinary aquaporin-2 may reflect the levels and/or activity of aquaporin-2 in the apical plasma membrane of the collecting duct. Analysis of urinary aquaporin-2 concentrations shows acute or long-term changes of the protein in a number of clinical conditions associated with water balance disorders. In that sense, low aquaporin-2 expression has been described in forms of nephrogenic diabetes insipidus (*e.g.* hypokalemia, hypercalcemia, lithium therapy, post-obstructive polyuria) as a mechanism for the inability of the kidney to concentrate urine in these conditions. In the pregnant rat, up-regulation of aquaporin-2 expression and aquaporin-2 trafficking was described. Administration of the V_2 receptor antagonist in pregnant rats suppressed the increase in aquaporin-2 mRNA and aquaporin-2 protein levels despite normal levels of plasma vasopressin thus suggesting that in pregnancy the up-regulation of aquaporin-2 contributes to water retention in part through a V_2 receptor-mediated effect. In addition, vasopressin-independent factors (such as oxytocin) may be important for this up-regulation.

Likewise, in pregnant women, up-regulation of aquaporin-2 expression and enhanced urinary protein levels have been substantially documented (Frokier et al., 1998); accordingly, this effect on aquaporin-2 is reversed by a V_2 receptor antagonist (Schrier, 2010). In a study of healthy pregnant primiparas, urinary aquaporin-2 excretion, plasma oxytocin and atrial natriuretic peptide but not plasma AVP levels were significantly higher in all three trimesters of pregnancy compared to age-matched non-pregnant women (Buemi, 2001) thus suggesting possible effects of an AVP-independent factor to stimulate renal aquaporin-2 expression during pregnancy.

In healthy adults, AVP circulates in an unbound state and equilibrates within minutes between plasma and the extracellular fluid. Its concentration in these compartments decreases with an average half-time of approximately 20 minutes. Normally, AVP is clearanced by the kidney or degraded by the liver; only a small quantity of AVP is taken up and stored by the platelets. During pregnancy, the increased AVP secretion is countered by a 3-fold to 6-fold increase in the metabolic clearance rate of vasopressin which is due to an enzyme, the vasopressinase. Vasopressinase is a plasmatic leucyl-cystinyl-aminopeptidase that degrades both AVP and oxytocin produced by the syncytiotrophoblast of the placenta. Because the placental trophoblastic mass increases about 1000-fold from 6 to 24 weeks of gestation, plasma vasopressinase levels may be 20-fold higher by the third trimester of pregnancy (Soule et al., 1995). Aside to vasopressinase, another enzyme of placental origin, leucine-aminopeptidase (oxytocinase) appears to contribute to AVP degradation during pregnancy. Plasma concentrations of leucine-aminopeptidase gradually increase during pregnancy until delivery, acting as an anti-uterotonic agent by degrading uterotonic peptides. Recently, preeclampsia was associated to low leucine-aminopeptidase levels (Landau et al., 2010). The accelerated AVP degradation resolves about 40 days post-delivery. Despite the increase in the clearance of AVP due to vasopressinase activity, in normal pregnancies, AVP levels remain unchanged thus suggesting a compensatory increase in synthesis and release. Nevertheless, it has to be pointed out that these adaptations are of no particular clinical relevance unless a pathological process is present.

Genetically AVP-deficient homozygous Brattleboro (BB) rats suffer from severe diabetes insipidus. The pregnant BB rat may serve as an animal model of central diabetes insipidus associated to pregnancy. Early studies have shown that the osmotic threshold for AVP during pregnancy is lower in both BB rats and controls and that, in the homozygous animal, chronic vasopressin treatment increased urine osmolality less compared with virgins (Barron et al., 1985). Nevertheless, the model does not apply to true gestational diabetes insipidus since this is induced by enhanced vasopressinase activity and metabolic AVP clearance. Besides AVP, oxytocin and relaxin may play a role in controlling water balance during physiological pregnancy. BB rats were found to significantly concentrate their urine upon severe dehydration, and the plasma level of oxytocin was found to be about 6-fold higher under these circumstances (Edwards & LaRochelle, 1984). An antidiuretic effect of oxytocin was evidenced in both normal individuals and central diabetes insipidus. Oxytocin has an affinity for the V_2 receptor two orders magnitude lower compared to that of 1-desamino-8-D-arginine (DDAVP). However, in a small study of healthy and diabetic men, oxytocin infusion resulted in decreased urine outflow and free water clearance and increased urine osmolality and aquaporin-2 urinary excretion (Koo et al., 2003) thus suggesting that, in man, the antidiuretic effect of oxytocin may be mediated by regulation of aquaporin-2 levels in the collecting duct.

Relaxin is characterized as a pregnancy-related hormone secreted by the corpus luteum involved as a key player in maternal systemic and renal vasodilatation during pregnancy, as revealed by the vasodilatation obtained in non-pregnant rats in response to intravenous relaxin administration. In human, emerging evidence suggests that the effect of relaxin is mediated by the relaxin/insulin-like family peptide 1 receptor, RFXP1, through a Gα-protein coupled to phosphatidylinositol-3kinase/Akt (protein kinase B)-dependent phosphorylation and activation of endothelial nitric oxide synthase to induce nitric oxide synthesis and, hence, important vasodilatation (Conrad, 2011).

4. Etiology and clinical presentation of pregnancy-related diabetes insipidus

4.1 Etiology of polyuria in pregnancy

Table 1 depicts potential causes of polyuria in pregnant women.

Solute Diuresis	Water Diuresis
Diabetes mellitus	Primary polyuria
Salt-losing tubulopathy	Diabetes insipidus
Saline loading	Hyperkalemia
Post-obstructive diuresis	Hypercalcemia
Osmotic iatrogenic diuresis	Primary or secondary tubulopathies
	Sickle cell anemia

Table 1. Causes of polyuria in pregnancy (adapted after Barbey et al., 2010).

Etiologic characterization of diabetes insipidus during pregnancy is complex and, in some cases, difficult to ascertain to one or the other related clinical conditions. Should diabetes predate pregnancy, in either overt or sub-clinical form, any disorder causing AVP-deficiency or AVP-resistance has to be taken into account. On the other hand, pregnancy itself may prone to development of pathological conditions of inadequate AVP synthesis or action, usually in a transient form during pregnancy and postpartum, but, occasionally, persisting thereafter. In synthesis, diabetes insipidus during pregnancy may reveal itself as:

- *Pre-gestational diabetes insipidus*, either central (AVP-deficient) or nephrogenic (AVP-resistant)
- *Latent (sub-clinical) central or nephrogenic diabetes insipidus*, unmasked by both increased vasopressinase activity and diminished renal responsiveness to vasopressin (Iwasaki et al., 1991)
- *True gestational diabetes insipidus*, as
    - *Transient gestational diabetes insipidus* which manifests in pregnancy and usually resolves 3-6 weeks after delivery. Multiple pregnancy acts as a risk factor. Transient gestational diabetes insipidus may be associated with preeclampsia, acute fatty liver disease or HELLP syndrome, or unmask prevalent liver disease such as in

hemochromatosis (Krysiak et al., 2010). As abovementioned, an underlying sub-clinical deficiency in AVP may also be involved in some, if not all, patients.

- *Recurrent diabetes insipidus of pregnancy* due to increased vasopressinase activity has been reported in subsequent pregnancies in several women. Both transient and recurrent gestational diabetes insipidus are vasopressin-resistant but respond well to desmopressin (DDAVP).
- *Transient, vasopressin- and DDAVP-resistant gestational diabetes insipidus* which is a consequence of the physiological increase in the concentration of prostaglandin E_2 in the kidney during gestation leading to inhibition of AVP action at the level of its receptor (Jin-No et al., 1998)

- *Postpartum diabetes insipidus* (*i.e.* lymphocytic hypophysitis, pituitary apoplexy, histiocytosis X, pituitary tumor, Sheehan's syndrome). Even though these pathological conditions clearly predominate within the first year after birth (postpartum period), concomitance with pregnancy is not excluded in any of them, except for Sheehan's syndrome.

In rare cases, gestational diabetes insipidus may develop as nephrogenic form manifested in pregnancy and complicated by preeclampsia (Goodman et al., 1984; Korbet et al., 1985). Diabetes insipidus may persist postpartum or may be a transient latent form of the disease.

4.2 Clinical features of pregnancy-related diabetes insipidus, and associated conditions

Clinical presentation of pregnancy-related diabetes insipidus is usually acute with symptoms developing in a few days. An abrupt change in the voiding pattern during the last trimester of pregnancy manifesting as hypotonic polyuria, and excessive water intake represent the hallmark of the disease. Fatigue, nausea, weight loss, and reduced skin turgor may be seen. Women in whom diabetes insipidus is associated to a more complex morbid status may present additional symptoms and clinical signs.

4.2.1 Pregnancy-related liver disease

Pregnancy-related liver disease comprises a large spectrum of liver disturbances specifically to pregnancy, with variable outcome potential. While liver dysfunction is transient and usually mild in *hyperemesis gravidarum* and intra-hepatic cholestasis of pregnancy, women with acute fatty liver disease or HELLP syndrome are at high risk to concomitantly develop preeclampsia and a less favorable prognosis. Differential diagnosis between pregnancy-related liver disease and preexistent or simultaneous hepatic disorder unrelated to pregnancy is mandatory and sometimes difficult.

Nevertheless, rarely, liver biopsy is employed as an ultimate differential diagnosis tool. Association of *de novo* diabetes insipidus with liver injury in pregnant women is suggested by polyuria and polydipsia syndrome and epigastric pain, nausea, vomiting, pruritus and jaundice. At least in some patients, acute fatty liver disease can be considered as an atypical form of preeclampsia because 30-40% of women with acute fatty liver also develop preeclampsia. In that sense, onset of diabetes insipidus in patients with acute fatty liver may highly indicate the likelihood of preeclampsia. Hence, early delivery and supportive care may considerably improve the overall prognosis of these individuals. Pathogenesis of diabetes insipidus in pregnant women with acute fatty liver can be easily explained by enhanced vasopressinase activity subsequent to liver dysfunction. Commonly, diabetes insipidus responds well to DDAVP therapy and spontaneously resolves with delivery or may persist postpartum for another few weeks.

Recently, it has been found that acute fatty liver of pregnancy is associated with a defect of long-chain 3-hydroxyacyl coenzyme A dehydrogenase in the fetus with c1528G>C point mutation as the main cause (Guttiérez Junquera et al., 2009). Therefore, genetic testing can be taken into consideration in both the mother and the fetus.

Association of advanced hepatocytolysis, hemolysis and thrombocytopenia gives birth to the HELLP syndrome, one component of systemic preeclampsia and eclampsia, often conjoined with diabetes insipidus, hypertension and cerebral edema. HELLP syndrome occurs in 10-20% of pregnancies with severe preeclampsia. The majority of cases (70%) develop in advanced pregnancy, between the 27th and 37th gestational week, and seldom later; the reminder within 48 hours after delivery, usually in women who developed proteinuria, hypertension, edema and excessive weight gain prior to delivery.

Recent studies hypothesized genetic predisposition as a risk factor for HELLP syndrome, mainly under the form of various disturbances in the process of blood coagulation. Therefore, some clinical studies investigated the association between hereditary thrombophilia and HELLP syndrome but results remain controversial (Ganzevoort et al., 2007; Larciprete et al., 2010). Several reports confirmed statistically higher incidence of antithrombin-III deficiency in patients with HELLP syndrome (Larciprete et al., 2010; Dogan et al., 2011). Apparently, women with elevated antiphospholipid antibodies titers are at risk to develop severe preeclampsia and HELLP syndrome (Heilmann et al., 2011).

Onset of HELLP syndrome is within days or weeks with headache, visual symptoms, malaise, nausea and vomiting and fluctuating abdominal pain. Most symptoms exacerbate during night. Para-clinical investigations will exhibit proteinuria, low hemoglobin levels and increased serum lactate dehydrogenase (LDH) concentrations to attest for onset of *microangiopathic hemolytic anemia* (Haram et al., 2009) in these patients. Elevated levels of liver enzymes (ASAT, ALAT and α-glutathione-S-transferase-a1) are documented. Thrombocytopenia is the result of subsequent increased platelet consumption and, thus, platelet turnover. If diabetes insipidus is present, hypernatremia, hemoconcentration and diminished urine/plasma osmolality ratio is expected. Table 2 summarizes the diagnosis criterions of HELLP syndrome according to the two major current definition systems.

	Mississippi Classification Criteria	*Tennessee Classification Criteria*
HELLP Syndrome	Platelet count ≤50 x 10^9/L AST or ALT ≥70 IU/L LDH ≥600 IU/L	Platelet count ≤100 x 10^9/L AST ≥70 IU/L LDH ≥600 IU/L

Table 2. Current diagnosis criteria for the HELLP syndrome.

Based on the platelet count, the Mississippi system categorizes the disorder into class 1 HELLP (table 2) and class 2 HELLP syndromes (*i.e.* platelet count ≤100 x 10^9/L and >50 x 10^9/L, serum liver enzymes ≥70 IU/L and serum LDH ≥600 IU/L). In addition, class 3 HELLP syndrome is defined according to Mississippi classification as platelet count ≤150 x 10^9/L and >100 x 10^9/L, serum liver enzymes ≥40 IU/L and serum LDH concentration ≥600 IU/L (Martin et al., 1999). Class 3 HELLP syndrome is considered a transitional group.

The clinical significance of HELLP syndrome is based upon severe maternal and fetal/neonatal complications that may occur in affected pregnancies. Biochemical abnormalities associated with increased risk of maternal complications consist of serum LDH levels >1400 IU/L, serum AST >150 IU/L, serum ALT >100 IU/L and serum uric acid levels >7.8 mg% (Magann & Martin, 1999). In the mother, life-threatening complications are *abruptio placentae,* disseminated intravascular coagulation, cerebral or brain stem hemorrhage, cerebral edema and spontaneous rupture of subcapsular liver hematoma. Purtscher-like retinopathy can result in permanent visual loss (Stewart et al., 2007).

Newborns from women with HELLP syndrome delivered before the 32th to 34th gestational week are at risk for intrauterine growth restriction, cardiovascular (*i.e.* persisting *ductus arteriosus*) and respiratory complications, and perinatal death due to prematurity, *abruptio placentae* or cerebral hemorrhage (*i.e.* caused by neonatal thrombocytopenia). Notably, complications in the newborn appear to be rather related to prematurity than to HELLP syndrome itself.

In women developing HELLP syndrome after the 34th week of pregnancy, vaginal delivery is the method of choice. Before the 34th gestational week, a single course of 12 mg betamethasone twice, 24 hours apart, is recommended to induce lung maturation. Repeated glucocorticoid courses may be more effective; however, they may lead to fetal growth restriction and prolonged adrenal suppression. High-dose dexamethasone treatment has been proposed as an alternative to improve maternal outcome, especially before 27th week of pregnancy, but there is no evidence of benefits compared to immediate delivery and thus should be individually addressed (Fonseca et al., 2005; Haram et al., 2009).

4.2.2 Lymphocytic (autoimmune) hypophysitis

Lymphocytic hypophysitis is a rare inflammatory disorder of the pituitary gland thought to have an autoimmune basis with predilection for women during the postpartum period and the late stage of pregnancy. Although lymphocytic hypophysitis should be always considered in the differential diagnosis of pituitary masses and/or pituitary insufficiency in women who are pregnant or in the early postpartum period, a definitive diagnosis of the disease requires pituitary biopsy. Nevertheless, a presumptive diagnosis of lymphocytic (autoimmune) hypophysitis is possible based on a history of gestational or postpartum pituitary insufficiency, rapid development of hypopituitarism in up to 75-80% of cases with early loss of adrenocorticotrophic hormone (ACTH) and TSH, and imagistic appearance of the pituitary gland and stalk including variable enlargement of the hypophysis with homogenous appearance and intact sella floor. Cystic appearance of the pituitary gland on magnetic resonance imaging (MRI), although rare, is not excluded in patients with autoimmune hypophysitis (Flanagan et al., 2002). In hypophysitis, the pituitary stalk is thickened but not displaced, an aspect that is opposed to the MRI of the displaced hypophyseal stalk that is described in macroadenomas with supra-sellar enlargement. A strong, homogenous enhancement of the anterior pituitary after gadolinium infusion, even though suggests inflammation, is not specific enough to differentiate between hypophysitis on one hand and pituitary adenoma on the other hand.

Autoimmune inflammation of the pituitary gland presents commonly as lymphocytic adenohypophysitis. The clinical presentation of autoimmune adenohypophysitis includes headache, pituitary insufficiency and central diabetes insipidus. Visual disturbances comprise visual field defects due to compression of the optic chiasm and diplopia due to compression of III, IV and VI cranial nerves by parasellar expansion of the autoimmune inflammatory process towards the cavernous sinus. Diabetes insipidus may be a component of pure lymphocytic adenohypophysitis because of inhibition of the axonal transport of

AVP by swelling of the *pars tuberalis* of the adenophypophysis which covers the infundibulum anterolaterally. From the clinical viewpoint, diabetes insipidus can be masked by coexistence of glucocorticoid deficiency in lymphocytic adenohypophysitis which is associated with stimulation of ADH release and aquaporin-2 synthesis (Caturegli et al., 2005) and is often revealed by glucocorticoid hormones replacement therapy. Long-term imagistic observation of few cases with a medical history of lymphocytic hypophysitis during pregnancy suggested that this clinical condition may evolve with pituitary atrophy and empty sella. Hence, it is believed that at least some cases with postpartum pituitary insufficiency (even Sheehan's syndrome) and empty sella may actually include lymphocytic adenohypophysitis (Ishihara et al., 1996).

Rarely, autoimmune inflammation of the pituitary gland may be limited to the posterior pituitary lobe and infundibular stem and termed lymphocytic infundibulo-hypophysitis. Lymphocytic infundibulo-hypophysitis has been reported as a cause of central diabetes insipidus in the postpartum period (VanHavenbergh et al., 1996). On MRI, infundibulo-hypophysitis is suspected on enlargement of the posterior pituitary lobe and thickening of the pituitary stalk greater than 3 mm at the level of the median eminence of the hypothalamus (Caturegli et al., 2005). Although loss of physiological T1 hyper-intensity in the posterior pituitary is suggestive, specificity of this aspect is low.

4.2.3 Pituitary apoplexy

Hemorrhagic or ischemic pituitary apoplexy is a rare neuro-endocrine emergency with a potentially severe outcome resulting even in hyponatremic coma and death. The main clinical symptoms are thunderclap headache, nausea and vomiting, fever, loss of consciousness, ophtalmoplegia, visual field impairment, monocular blindness and neck stiffness (meningeal irritation). The diagnosis is most challenging in apparently healthy subjects (Georgescu et al., 2009) in whom neurological complications such as stroke, meningitis, diffuse subarachnoid hemorrhage or optic tract hemorrhage may develop. Occasionally, pituitary apoplexy may present as isolated unilateral or bilateral IIIrd or VIth nerve palsy.

In most cases, pituitary apoplexy complicates the evolution of previously diagnosed adenomas. In a retrospective review of 28 cases with pituitary adenoma, 14% of patients were incidentally diagnosed after pituitary apoplexy (Dekkers et al., 2007) and in a follow-up of 42 patients with incidentally found non-functioning pituitary adenoma, apoplexy complicated the natural course of the disease in 9.5% of cases. On the other hand, in a large series of 45 cases of subjects with pituitary apoplexy, only 18% were known to have pituitary adenoma at presentation (Sibal et al., 2004). Likewise, in a larger series of 62 patients with this clinical condition, 81% of subjects had no previous medical history suggesting pituitary tumor (Semple et al., 2005).

Pituitary apoplexy in pregnancy and postpartum is even more rarely encountered with less than 50 cases reported in the medical literature. Occasionally, spontaneous abortion develops during the follow-up (Krull et al., 2010). To confirm diagnosis, pituitary hormones evaluation and MRI assessment of the hypothalamus-pituitary region is mandatory. MRI is revealing a sellar mass with fluid level or central component suggesting hemorrhage. Extrasellar expansion is common resulting in pituitary stalk displacement and optic chiasm compression.

Pituitary insufficiency of various degrees follows the onset of pituitary apoplexy. Note worthily, the association of pituitary apoplexy with permanent or transient diabetes insipidus is rather rare, irrespective of gender and physiological status; in two larger studies, of 62 and 40 patients, respectively, only 8% of subjects developed AVP deficiency (Semple et al., 2005; Lubina et al., 2005). Artery surgery, other major surgery, pregnancy, gamma knife irradiation, anticoagulant therapy, and coagulopathy secondary to liver failure were identified as precipitating factors for pituitary apoplexy. Specific information on the prevalence of diabetes insipidus in women developing pituitary apoplexy in pregnancy and postpartum is not yet available.

With except of cases developing compression of the optic chiasm or severe neurological status, pituitary apoplexy in pregnancy should be treated preferably conservatively with high-dose glucocorticoid therapy and hormone replacement therapy including AVP- or DDAVP medication if diabetes insipidus is diagnosed. Monitoring by MRI is recommended. In advanced gestation delivery is preferred.

4.2.4 Sheehan's syndrome

Sheehan's syndrome describes postpartum pituitary necrosis; however, the exact pathogenic mechanism of the syndrome is not well understood because such endocrine abnormalities are not obvious in most women with severe hemorrhage in pregnancy and delivery. Although not a typical feature of Sheehan's syndrome, early postpartum diabetes insipidus may accompany postpartum pituitary necrosis in about 5% of cases and even more when systematically looked for. In a study on posterior pituitary function in 26 women with Sheehan's syndrome by both water deprivation and 5% hypertonic saline infusion test, partial diabetes insipidus was diagnosed in 29.6% of patients (Atmaca et al., 2007). Likewise, plasma AVP measurements after the 5% hypertonic saline infusion test in women with postpartum hypopituitarism but absent polyuria revealed, in 10 of 12 patients, the presence of various degrees of subnormal AVP responses to the increase in plasma osmolality (Iwasaki et al., 1989). Higher osmotic threshold for thirst perception was described in Sheehan's syndrome patients in comparison to controls; thus, besides AVP insufficiency, ischemic damage of the thirst center may contribute to increased osmotic threshold for the onset of thirst in Sheehan's syndrome (Atmaca et al., 2007).

Occasionally, in women with pre-pregnancy diagnosis of Sheehan's syndrome, latent central diabetes insipidus may became manifest during pregnancy (Briet et al., 1998) to be corrected with vasopressin therapy. Water metabolism disturbances in patients with Sheehan's syndrome depend on several factors such as the degree of pituitary damage, the time of onset since the pituitary injury, association of co-morbidities and/or concomitant medication. Emerging evidence shows that Sheehan's syndrome with or without diabetes insipidus is increasingly reported in association with antiphospholipid syndrome (Mehdi et al., 2011). In addition, in advanced pregnancy, contribution of enhanced vasopressinase activity to disturbed water balance should be considered and is suggested by incomplete response of polyuria and polydipsia to vasopressin but adequate control by desmopressin. Exceptionally, postpartum Sheehan's syndrome may evolve to acute renal failure.

5. Impact of pregnancy-related diabetes insipidus on maternal and fetal health

Pre-pregnancy confirmed, therapeutically controlled diabetes insipidus has normally no significant impact on pregnancy outcome and health status of the fetus. On the contrary, gestational diabetes insipidus is potentially related to a series of maternal-fetal complications, of maximum severity in cases associated with HELLP syndrome and pre-eclampsia. Maternal complications may include severe hypernatremia, eclampsia, hepatic insufficiency and disseminated intravascular coagulation. In several cases, premature delivery of the fetus avoids fetal hypoxia and intrauterine fetal death (Wiser et al., 2008).

Generally, transient diabetes insipidus recovers about 4-6 weeks after delivery. Rarely, permanent central diabetes insipidus with or without definitive pituitary insufficiency of various degrees may occur in the mother, depending on the underlying clinical condition of pregnancy-related diabetes.

Gestational diabetes insipidus may associate *in utero* fetal complications such as oligohydramnios or polyhydramnios. Rapid-onset polyhydramnios and fetal polyuria were recently described by Weinberg (Weinberg et al., 2010) in a singleton pregnancy developing transient third trimester gestational diabetes insipidus in the mother. Nevertheless, the mechanism of fetal polyuria remains elusive in this case. The authors' speculated on either maternal over-hydration or an effect on fetal vasopressin of the increased maternal vasopressinase, for which transplacental passage has been described.

6. Fetal disorders/conditions associated with disturbances in ADH production or activity and their repercussions on the pregnancy course

Both AVP and oxytocin are synthesized by the hypothalamic supraoptic and paraventricular nuclei during the first weeks of fetal life. AVP is found in high concentrations in fetal plasma and neonate umbilical cord blood and thought to be involved in blood pressure regulation. The main stimulus of AVP release in the fetus is hypoxia but also hypotension, acidosis and hypercarbia may play a role. Aquaporin-2 metabolism in the fetus and neonate is not fully understood. Researches in both preterm and at term infants suggested that in early postnatal life aquaporin-2 urinary levels cannot serve as a marker of AVP renal action and renal capacity to concentrate urine (Nyul et al., 2002; Zelenina et al., 2006) although opposing results were reported (Iacobelli et al., 2006). Nevertheless, in the same studies urinary aquaporin-2 concentrations correlated adequately with the overall maturity of tubular renal function and decreased in conditions of impaired kidney activity. In the fetus and newborn, diabetes insipidus is a rare disorder with a complex pathogenesis (table 3).

Most cases of central diabetes insipidus are secondary to a known etiology while defective AVP action is often related to a pathological condition and/or specific medication in the pregnant mother.

Clinically, diabetes insipidus may be suspected in newborns presenting during the first days of life with polyuria and weight loss, and is confirmed by hypernatremia, high plasmatic osmolality and low urine osmolality and a good response to desmopressin. Nevertheless, diagnosis during the neonatal period may be difficult because of frequent lack of polyuria due to the decreased renal glomerular filtration that exists during the neonatal period. The increase in the glomerular filtration rate thereafter unmasks the later polyuria. Moreover, the low osmolarity of the breast milk may mask specific features of diabetes insipidus in neonates that are exclusively breastfed. The disorder may be suspected in infants with unexplained fever, irritability, lack of weight gain, hypernatremia. Often, the child can be calmed with water but not with milk. Rapid management is required to prevent potentially lethal complications such as intracranial bleeding and renal vein thrombosis.

Central diabetes insipidus	Nephrogenic diabetes insipidus
Perinatal asphyxia	Medication (in the mother) (*e.g.* lithium, angiotensin-converting enzyme inhibitors, angiotensin type 1 receptor blockers)
Intracranial hemorrhage (e.g. vitamin K deficiency)	Familial or sporadic congenital nephrogenic diabetes insipidus
Infection (e.g. congenital toxoplasmosis, congenital cytomegalovirus infection, meningitis: streptococcal, meningococcal, listeria meningitis, brain abscess)	
Congenital defects in the brain/pituitary morphogenesis (e.g. pituitary agenesis/hypogenesis, septo-optic dysplasia, holoprosencephaly, congenital nasal pyriform aperture stenosis, cleft lip/palate, meningomyelocele, hydrocephalus, facial diplegia (Mobius syndrome), Delleman syndrome, Kabuki syndrome etc.	
Cranio-cerebral trauma	
Intracranial tumors (e.g. teratoma, craniopharyngioma)	
Cysts	
Familial central diabetes insipidus	
Wolfram syndrome*	

Table 3. Etiology and pathogenesis of diabetes insipidus in the fetus and neonate.*onset of diabetes insipidus is confirmed after the age of 3 month.

6.1 Central diabetes insipidus in the fetus and neonate

Congenital isolated central diabetes insipidus may be of idiopathic nature (Bianchi, 2010) or due to various underlying pathological states (Table 3). Idiopathic central diabetes insipidus has been particularly reported in preterm very low birth weight infants (Stapleton & Di Geronimo, 2000). Central diabetes insipidus appears as a component of congenital anomalies, in particular midline developmental defects or genetic syndromes, of which the most important are represented by:

- midline craniofacial malformations (holoprosencephaly)
- septo-optic dysplasia (De Morsier's syndrome) is a complex disorder that consists in incomplete development of midline cranial structures such as hypoplasia/aplasia of the optic nerves, hypoplasia/absence of the *septum pellucidum* and/or pituitary hypoplasia/aplasia, with isolated or combined pituitary hormone deficiencies including AVP deficiency and in particular growth hormone deficiency. *HESX1* gene mutations have been associated with septo-optic dysplasia.
- Delleman syndrome associating somatic changes such as macrocephaly, micrognathia, anophtalmia, cleft lip and palate, *cutis aplasia*, diabetes insipidus and panhypopituitarism (Leichtman et al., 1994)
- Kabuki syndrome, a multiple malformation disorder caused by mutations in the *MLL2* gene (Ng et al., 2010), a histone methyltransferase ubiquitary expressed among adult

human tissues; affected individuals may present with strabismus, long palpebral fissures, large ears, cardiac and immunological anomalies, dwarfism and mental retardation. Diabetes insipidus may develop.

In fact, any severe defect of brain development can be associated to diabetes insipidus due to alterations in pituitary embryogenesis.

- Pituitary agenesis/hypogenesis with absence of the pituitary stalk
- Wolfram syndrome or DIDMOAD with an autosomal recessive transmission pattern, which combines diabetes insipidus, diabetes mellitus, optic atrophy, deafness, atonia of the bladder, hydronephrosis, neurological and gastrointestinal anomalies, hypogonadotropic hypogonadism and depression. In contrast to diabetes mellitus which develops early, even during neonatal life, diabetes insipidus appears in up to 75% of affected individuals, with a peak incidence at age 15 (range 3 months - 40 years). Desmopressin treatment adequately controls diabetes insipidus. The gene involved in most Wolfram syndrome cases is called *WFS1* and located in the chromosomal region 4p16.1. The WFS1 protein, also known as wolframin, appears to be involved in cell cycle regulation and apoptosis. Recently, another mutation associated with the *WSF2* locus on chromosome 4 has been identified in patients suffering from Wolfram syndrome (Amr et al., 2010).
- Familial central diabetes insipidus may be transmitted autosomal dominant, autosomal recessive or X-linked with variable penetrability.

Congenital toxoplasmosis may result in central diabetes insipidus. In that case, the serum and cerebrospinal fluid samples of the patient test positive for toxoplasmosis. Alternatively, etiology is suggested by cranial computed tomography revealing obstructive hydrocephalus and cranial disseminated calcifications. Anterior pituitary insufficiency is occasionally cited in neonates with congenital toxoplasmosis with central adrenal insufficiency and central hypothyroidism (Siahanidou et al., 2006). One case of prolonged fever, attributed to hypothalamic dysfunction (hypothalamic fever) has been reported in association to diabetes insipidus in a newborn diagnosed with congenital toxoplasmosis (Siahanidou et al., 2006).

Tumors of the hypothalamus-pituitary region may account for onset of central fetal/neonatal diabetes insipidus. Neonatal craniopharyngioma has been repeatedly reported as a suprasellar tumor with partially cystic appearance in MRI and variable outcome after radical neurosurgery (Müller et al., 2000). Arachnoid cysts with suprasellar localization may manifest with pituitary insufficiency and central diabetes insipidus when the cyst reaches a sufficient size. In Langerhans cell histiocytosis early infiltration of the hypothalamus and pituitary stalk causes central diabetes insipidus. Combined Langerhans cell histiocytosis and DiGeorge Syndrome displaying multisystemic involvement of Letterer-Siewe disease at birth has been reported (Levendoglu et al., 1996). Transiently, central diabetes insipidus in the neonate is described in association with hypotonia, dysmorphism and marked speech delay due to 22q13 deletion syndrome (Barakat et al., 2004).

6.2 Nephrogenic diabetes insipidus in the fetus and neonate

Congenital nephrogenic either sporadic or familial diabetes insipidus is caused in 90% of cases by X-linked transmitted mutations in the AVP receptor 2 gene that encodes for the AVP type 2 receptor. Until now, five types of molecular defects in the protein synthesis or action have been described. The other 10% of cases result from mutations in the aquaporin-2 gene. Autosomal recessive inheritance of the mutation results in proteins that remain

trapped in the endoplasmic reticulum and are rapidly degraded, whereas autosomal dominant inheritance results in synthesis of structurally normal proteins but inable to ensure intracellular transport within the tubular renal cell. In few cases of congenital nephrogenic diabetes insipidus neither the AVP gene nor the aquaporin-2 gene are affected.
Note worthily, nephrogenic diabetes insipidus in the fetus may be a result of maternal medication such as lithium, angiotensin-converting enzyme inhibitors or angiotensin type 1 receptor blockers. Lithium is commonly used in the treatment of psychiatric disorders, specifically bipolar depression. Lithium causes polyhydramnios from fetal diabetes insipidus *in utero*. Clinical presentation of infants with *in utero* lithium exposure comprises transient neuro-developmental deficiencies such as hypoglycemia, hyperbilirubinemia, hypotonia, respiratory distress syndrome, cyanosis, lethargy, and weak suck and Moro reflexes in the neonatal period. Additionally, large-for-gestational age and prematurity, Ebstein's anomaly, cardiovascular toxicity and endocrine complications have been reported. Of endocrine disorders, newborns are at risk to develop nephrogenic diabetes insipidus and thyroid dysfunction (Kozma et al., 2005).
Alternatively, other congenital tubulopathies can associate a partial defect in the capacity to concentrate urine and usually present with a low degree of polyuria (*e.g.* Bartter syndrome, Fanconi syndrome, nephronophtisis, polycystic kidneys, obstructive nephropathy, nephritis, renal insufficiency).

7. Diagnostic challenges in pregnancy-related diabetes insipidus

Whatever etiology of diabetes insipidus, the main feature consists of excretion of high amounts of dilute, flavorless, hypotonic urine. Irrespective of the pathogenesis of the disorder (*i.e.* central, gestational or nephrogenic diabetes insipidus), a primary deficiency in urinary concentration will result in a rise of urine flow that produces a slight (1% to 2%) decrease in body water and a commensurate rise in basal plasma osmolality and sodium. Therefore, high urine output with low urine specific gravity (<1005) and low urine osmolality (50-300 mOsm/kg) in the presence of normal or elevated sodium (148 mmol/l) or plasma osmolality strongly suggests diabetes insipidus. Exclusion of other causes of polyuria such as diabetes mellitus, renal failure, hypokalemia, hypercalcemia and tubular renal acidosis is made by determination of fasting glucose and oral glucose tolerance test, urea, creatinine, creatinine clearance and electrolytes in blood and urine. Adrenal function tests, thyroid tests and basal and dynamic tests of pituitary function should be considered.
The practice of relating plasma to urine osmolality is useful; it can quickly differentiate diabetes insipidus from parenteral fluid excess. The urine osmolality is a measure of the concentration of the urine and is determined by AVP concentration. In a hypernatremic patient, a urine osmolality below that of the plasma suggests diabetes insipidus.
In contrast to women with primary polyuria, women with diabetes insipidus will not concentrate their urine osmolality during the water deprivation test. However, differential diagnosis from primary polydipsia may be difficult in women with partial AVP deficiency since fluid restriction can increase AVP secretion sufficiently to concentrate the urine. Additionally, the water deprivation test performed during pregnancy needs closed observation of the patient and may be problematic because the resulting plasma volume may lead to important dehydration and may increase the risk of utero-placental insufficiency. In this case diagnostic tests may be limited to measurement of urine and plasma osmolality and AVP or DDAVP administration.

Partial or mild forms of diabetes insipidus, however, cannot be clearly differentiated by indirect tests. In these cases, plasma AVP measurement with a high sensitivity assay, before and after water deprivation or osmotic stimulation during infusion of hypertonic 5% saline increases diagnosis accuracy (Zerbe & Robertson, 1981). Using a nomogram, AVP remains low after hypertonic saline infusion in patients with cranial diabetes insipidus while it increases normally in relation to plasma osmolality in patients with primary polyuria. Pregnant women with pre-existing central diabetes insipidus will respond by increased urine osmolality after intranasal delivery of AVP or AVP injection, as will patients developing hypothalamus-pituitary disorders during pregnancy. In contrast, vasopressin resistance is well-described in transient or recurrent gestational diabetes insipidus due to vasopressinase, however, patients will adequately respond to DDAVP. If there is a normal response to AVP or DDAVP that is urine osmolality obtained 30–60 min after injection increases, nephrogenic diabetes insipidus can be ruled out. All pregnant women with diabetes insipidus of unclear etiology should undergo magnetic resonance imaging of the hypothalamus-pituitary region to establish coexistence of disorders that may have affected AVP-producing neurons.

Notably, differential diagnosis of diabetes insipidus in pregnant women without pre-dating disease may be challenging and, occasionally, certainty with regard to the etiopathogeny is obtained after delivery. However, it has to be kept in mind that persistence of polyuria and polydipsia more than 6 weeks postpartum questions the diagnosis of true gestational diabetes insipidus and needs re-evaluation of the case.

8. Therapy of diabetes insipidus in pregnancy and lactation

Once the diagnosis is established, close monitoring of vital signs, fetal status, fluid balance, body weight and renal function are essential. Fluid intake must approximate urine volume and other fluid losses. Many patients require parenteral treatment, which usually consists of 5% glucose and normal saline infusion. Vaginal delivery with regional analgesia or, in the case of cesarean section, spinal anesthesia, are the methods of choice.

Earlier pituitary extracts of AVP contained oxytocin and precipitated uterine contractions and preterm labor. Chlorpropamide can stimulate secretion of AVP and potentiate its effects but it can cause fetal hypoglycemia and neonatal diabetes insipidus.

Because AVP degradation by vasopressinase is initiated by clipping the first amino-acid of the hormone, whereas its analog called DDAVP (1-deamino-8-D-arginine vasopressin, desmopressin acetate) is devoid of the first amino acid of AVP, the treatment of choice in patients with pregnancy-related diabetes insipidus is DDAVP. In contrast to the naturally occurring hormone, arginine-vasopressin, DDAVP exhibits practically no pressor activity and a prolonged antidiuretic activity lasting from 8 to 12 h (Fjellestad-Paulsen et al., 1993). There are several routes of administration of DDAVP. In pregnancy, the intranasal, oral or sublingual routes are preferred (Table 4).

Intransal		*Oral*	*Sublingual (Melt)*
Spray	*Drops*	*Tablets*	*Tablets*
-	5 µg	100 µg	60 µg
10 µg	10 µg	200 µg	120 µg
20 µg	20 µg	400 µg	240 µg

Table 4. Dose comparison of different DDAVP (desmopressin acetate) formulations.

Decreased response to nasal DDAVP may occur during episodes of rhinitis. In these cases or when oral administration is not possible, and in the postoperative period, the parenteral form (4 μg/ml, intravenously, intramuscularly or subcutaneously) is preferred.
Experience with the use of DDAVP during pregnancy is increasing; it is safe for both the mother and the fetus. In fact, DDAVP appears not to cross the placenta within detectable limits (Ray et al., 2004). To be mentioned, however, there is large individual variation in the amplitude and duration of effect. Hence, doses have to be tailored individually for optimal efficacy.
Hyponatremia is reported to occur after first doses of DDAVP in patients who do not restricte oral water intake; therefore, desmopressin carries the potential hazard of dilutional hyponatremia if the patient continues to drink inappropriately despite persistent antidiuresis. Lower extremity edema and signs of water intoxication may develop in cases with excessive dosage.

9. Conclusion

Diabetes insipidus in pregnancy and postpartum is an endocrine disorder with potentially serious consequences on the maternal course of gestation and on fetal development and health when occurring in association with life-threatening clinical conditions such as preeclampsia, HELLP syndrome or pituitary insufficiency. Although described more than one hundred years ago, the disease is not fully understood from the pathophysiological point of view and appears to be under-diagnosed. Basically, most information available in this area of knowledge resulted from isolated case reports or case series reviews, while on the contrary few conclusions were drawn from systematic studies documenting disease prevalence and therapy. To improve knowledge in the diagnosis and multispecialty management of women with pregnancy-related diabetes insipidus and their offspring, further studies are warranted.

10. References

Aleksandrov, N.; Audibert, F.; Bedard, M.J.; Mahone, M.; Goffinet, F. & Kadoch, I.J. (2010). Gestational diabetes insipidus: a review of an underdiagnosed condition. *J Obstet Gynaecol Can*, Vol.32, No.3, (April, 2011), pp. 225-231, ISSN 1701-2163.

Momigliano, E. (1929). Diabete insipido e gravidanza. *Ann di Ostet e Ginec*, Vol.51, (1971), pp. 905-979, ISSN 0003-4657.

Bleakley, J. (1938). A case of diabetes insipidus and twin pregnancy. *Proc R Soc Med*, Vol.31, No.9, (March, 2011), pp. 1062-1064, ISSN 0035-9157.

Blotner, H. & Kunkel, P. (1942). Diabetes insipidus and pregnancy - report of two cases. *N Engl J Med*, Vol.227, No.8, (April, 2011), pp. 287-292, ISSN *0028-4793.*

Chellakooty, M.; Skibsted, L.; Skouby, S.O.; Andersson, A.M.; Petersen, J.H.; Main, K.M.; Skakkebaek, N.E. & Juul, A. (2002). Longitudinal study of serum placental GH in 455 normal pregnancies: correlation to gestational age, fetal gender, and weight. *J Clin Endocrinol Metab*, Vol.87, No.6, (April, 2011), pp. 2734-2739, ISSN 0021-972X.

Glinoer, D. (1997). The regulation of thyroid function in pregnancy: pathways of endocrine adaptation from physiology to pathology. *Endocr Rev*, Vol.18, (April, 2011), pp: 404-433, ISSN 0163-769.

Karaca, Z.; Tanriverdi, F.; Unluhizarci, K. & Kelestimur, F. (2010). Pregnancy and pituitary disorders. *Eur J Endocrinol,* Vol.162, No.3, (May, 2011), pp. 453-475, ISSN 0804-4643.

Kalantaridou, S.N.; Makrigiannakis, A.; Mastorakos, G. & Chrousos, G.P. (2003). Roles of reproductive corticotropin-releasing hormone. *Ann N Y Acad Sci,* Vol.997 (April, 2011), pp. 129-135, ISSN 0077-8923.

Schrier, R.W. & Briner, V.A. (1991). Peripheral arterial vasodilation hypothesis of sodium and water retention in pregnancy: implications for pathogenesis of preeclampsia-eclampsia. *Obstet Gynecol,* Vol.77 (May, 2011), pp. 632–639, ISSN 0029-7844.

Schrier, R.W. & Ohara, M. (2010). Dilemmas in human and rat pregnancy: proposed mechanisms relating to arterial vasodilation. *J Neuroendocrinol,* Vol.22, No.5 (May, 2011), pp. 400-406, ISSN 1365-2826.

Lindheimer, M.D. & Davison, J.M. (1995). Osmoregulation, the secretion of arginine vasopressin and its metabolism during pregnancy. *Eur J Endocrinol,* Vol.132, No.2, (May, 2011), pp. 133-143, ISSN 0804-4643.

Davison, J.M.; Shiells, E.A.; Philips, P.R. & Lindheimer, M.D. (1988). Serial evaluation of vasopressin release and thirst in human pregnancy. Role of human chorionic gonadotrophin in the osmoregulatory changes of gestation. *J Clin Invest,* Vol.81 (April, 2011), pp. 798-806, ISSN 0021-9738.

Schrier, R.W.; Ohara, M.; Rogachev, B.; Xu, L. & Knotek, M. (1998). Aquaporin-2 water channels and vasopressin antagonists in edematous disorders. *Mol Genet Metab,* Vol.65, (April, 2011), pp. 255–263, ISSN 1096-7192.

Frokiaer, J.; Marples, D.; Knepper, MA. & Nielsen, S. (1998). Pathophysiology of aquaporin-2 in water balance disorders. *Am J Med Sci,* Vol.316, No.5, (May, 2011), pp. 291-299, ISSN 0002-9629.

Buemi, M. (2001). Urinary excretion of aquaporin-2 water channel during pregnancy. *Cell Physiol Biochem,* Vol.11, (3-4, 2011), pp. 203-208, ISSN 1015-8987.

Soule, S.G.; Monson, J.P. & Jacobs, H.S. (1995). Transient diabetes insipidus in pregnancy: a consequence of enhanced placental clearance of arginine vasopressin. *Hum Reprod,* Vol.10, (May, 2011), pp. 3322–3324, ISSN 0268-1161.

Landau, R.; Laverrière, A.; Bischof, P.; Irion, O.; Morales, M. & Cohen, M. (2010). Alteration of circulating Placental Leucine Aminopeptidase (P-LAP) activity in preeclampsia. *Neuro Endocrinol Lett,* Vol.31, No.1, (February, 2011), pp. 63-66, ISSN 0172–780X.

Barron, W.M.; Dürr, J.; Stamoutsos, B.A. & Lindheimer, MD. (1985). Osmoregulation and vasopressin secretion during pregnancy in Brattleboro rats. *Am J Physiol,* Vol.248 (May, 2011), pp. 29-37, ISSN 0363-6135.

Edwards, B. & LaRochelle, FT Jr. (1984). Antidiuretic effect of endogenous oxytocin in dehydrated Brattleboro homozygous rats. *Am J Physiol,* Vol.247, (May, 2011), pp. 453–F465, ISSN 0363-6135.

Koo, K.W.; Jeon, U.S.; Kim, G.H.; Park, J.; Oh, Y.K.; Kim, Y.S.; Ahn, C.; Kim, S.; Kim S.Y.; Lee, J.S. & Han, J.S. (2003). Antidiuretic action of oxytocin is associated with increased urinary excretion of aquaporin-2. *Nephrol Dial Transpl,* Vol.19, No.10, (April, 2011), pp. 2480-2486, ISSN 0931- 0509.

Conrad, K.P. (2011). Emerging role of relaxin in the maternal adaptations to normal pregnancy: implications for preeclampsia. *Semin Nephrol,* Vol.31, No.1, (March, 2011), pp. 15-32 ISSN 0270-9295.

Barbey, F.; Bonny, O.; Rothuizen, L.; Gomez, F. & Burnier, M. (2003). A pregnant woman with de novo polyuria-polydipsia and elevated liver enzymes. *Nephrol Dial Transpl,* Vol.18, No.10, (April, 2011), pp. 2193-2196 ISSN 0931- 0509.

Iwasaki, Y.; Oiso, Y.; Kondo, K., Takagi, S.; Takatsuki, K.; Hasegawa, H.; Ishikawa, K.; Fujimura, Y.; Kazeto, S.; Tomita, A. (1991). Aggravation of subclinical diabetes insipidus during pregnancy. *N Engl J Med,* Vol.324, (May, 2011), pp:522-526, ISSN 0028-4793.

Krysiak. R.; Kobielusz-Gembala, I. & Okopien, B. (2010). Recurrent pregnancy-induced diabetes insipidus in a woman with hemochromatosis. *Endocr J,* Vol.57, No.12, (March, 2011), pp. 1023-1028, ISSN 0918-8959.

Jin-no, Y.; Kamiya, Y.; Okada, M.; Watanabe, O.; Ogasawara, M. & Fujinami, T. (1998). Pregnant woman with transient diabetes insipidus resistant to 1-desamino-8-D-arginine vasopressin. *Endocr J,* Vol.45, No.5, (March, 2011), pp. 693-696, ISSN 0918-8959.

Goodman, H.; Sachs, B.P.; Phillippe, M. & Moore, T. (1984). Transient, recurrent nephrogenic diabetes insipidus. *Am J Obstet Gynecol,* Vol.149, No.8, (April, 2011), pp. 910-912, ISSN 0002-9378.

Korbet, S.M.; Corwin, H.L. & Lewis, E.J. (1985). Transient nephrogenic diabetes insipidus associated with pregnancy. *Am J Nephrol,* Vol.5, No.6, (6, 2011), pp. 442-444 ISSN 0250-8095.

Gutiérrez Junquera, C.; Balmaseda, E.; Gil, E.; Martínez, A.; Sorli, M.; Cuartero, I.; Merinero, B.; Ugarte, M. (2009). Acute fatty liver of pregnancy and neonatal long-chain 3-hydroxyacyl-coenzyme A dehydrogenase (LCHAD) deficiency. *Eur J Pediatr,* Vol.168, No. 1, (May, 2011), pp. 103-106, ISSN 0340-6199.

Ganzevoort, W.; Rep, A.; De Vries, J.I.; Bonsel, G.J.; Wolf, H. & PETRA-Investigators. (2007). Relationship between thrombophilic disorders and type of severe early-onset hypertensive disorder of pregnancy. *Hypertens Pregnancy,* Vol.26, No.4, (March-April, 2011), pp. 433-445, ISSN 1064-1955.

Larciprete, G.; Rossi, F.; Deaibess, T.; Brienza, L.; Barbati, G.; Romanini, E.; Gioia, S. & Cirese, E. (2010). Double inherited thrombophilias and adverse pregnancy outcomes: fashion or science? *J Obstet Gynaecol Res,* Vol.35, No.5, (April, 2011), pp. 996-1002, ISSN 1341-8076.

Dogan, OO.; Simsek, Y.; Celen. S. & Danisman, N. (2011). Frequency of hereditary thrombophilia, anticoagulant activity, and homocysteine levels in patients with hemolysis, elevated liver functions and low thrombocyte count (HELLP) syndrome. *J Obstet Gynaecol Res,* URL: 10.1111/j.1447-0756.2010.01397, ISSN 1341-8076.

Heilmann, L.; Schorsch, M.; Hahn, T. & Fareed, J. (2011). Antiphospholipid syndrome and pre-eclampsia. *Semin Thromb Hemost,* Vol.37, No.2, (April, 2011), pp. 141-145, ISSN 0094-6176.

Haram, K.; Svendsen, E. & Abildgaard, U. (2009). The HELLP syndrome: clinical issues and management. A Review. *BMC Pregnancy Childbirth,* Vol.26, No.9, (April, 2011), pp. 8, ISSN 1471-2393.

Martin, J.N.Jr.; Rinehart, B.K.; May, W.L.; Magann, E.F.; Terrone, D.A. & Blake, P.G. (1999). The spectrum of severe preeclampsia: comparative analysis by HELLP (hemolysis, elevated liver enzyme levels, and low platelet count) syndrome classification. *Am J Obstet Gynecol,* Vol.180, No.6, (April, 2011), pp. 1373-1384, ISSN 0002-9378.

Magann, E.F. & Martin, J.N.Jr. (1999). Twelve steps to optimal management of HELLP syndrome. *Clin Obstet Gynecol,* Vol.42, (Jun, 2011), pp.532–550, ISSN 0009-9201.

Stewart, M.W.; Brazis, P.W.; Guier, C.P.; Thota, S.H. & Wilson, S.D. (2007). Purtscher-like retinopathy in a patient with HELLP syndrome. *Am J Ophthalmol,* Vol.143, No.5, (May, 2011), pp. 886-887, ISSN 0002-9394.

Fonseca, J.E.; Méndez, F.; Cataño, C. & Arias F. (2005). Dexamethasone treatment does not improve the outcome of women with HELLP syndrome: a double-blind, placebo-controlled, randomized clinical trial. *Am J Obstet Gynecol,* Vol.193, No.5, (April, 2011), pp. 1591-1598, ISSN 0002-9378.

Flanagan, D.E.; Ibrahim, A.E.; Ellison, D.W.; Armitage, M.; Gawne-Cain, M. & Lees, P.D. (2002). Inflammatory hypophysitis—the spectrum of disease. *Acta Neurochir (Wien),* Vol.144, (May, 2011), pp. 47–56, ISSN 0001-6268.

Caturegli, P.; Newschaffer C.; Olivi, A.; Pomper, M.G.; Burger, P.C. & Rose, N.R. (2005). Autoimmune hypophysitis *Endocr Rev,* Vol.26, No.5, (May, 2011), pp. 599-614, ISSN 0163-769X.

Ishihara, T.; Hino, M.; Kurahachi, H.; Kobayashi, H.; Kajikawa, M.; Moridera, K.; Ikekubo K. & Hattori, N. (1996). Long-term clinical course of two cases of lymphocytic adenohypophysitis. *Endocr J,* Vol.43, No.4, (March, 2011), pp. 433-440, ISSN 0918-8959.

VanHavenbergh, T.; Robberecht, W.; Wilm, G.; VanCalenbergh, F.; Goffin, J.; Dom, R.; Bouillon, R. & Plets, C. (1996). Lymphocytic infundibulohypophysitis presenting in the postpartum period: Case report. *Surg Neurol,* Vol.46, No.3, (December, 2009), pp. 280-284, ISSN 0090-3019.

Georgescu, C.E.; Ilie, I.; Moldovan, F.; Stan, H.; Albu, S.; & Duncea, I. (2010). Thunderclap headache caused by a pituitary non-functioning tumour presenting as spontaneous pituitary apoplexy. *Rom J Neurol,* Vol.IX, No.1, (March, 2011), pp. 33-37, ISSN 1843-8148.

Dekkers, O.M.; Hammer, S.; de Keizer, R.J.; Roelfsema, F.; Schutte, P.J.; Smith, J.W.; Romijn, J.A. & Pereira, A.M. (2007). The natural course of non-functioning pituitary macroadenomas. *Eur J Endocrinol,* Vol.156, No.2, (May, 2011), pp. 217-224, ISSN 0804-4643.

Sibal, L.; Ball, S.G.; Connolly, V.; James, R.A.; Kane, P.; Kelly, W.F.; Kendall-Taylor, P.; Mathias, D.; Perros, P.; Quinton, R. & Vaidya, B. (2004). Pituitary apoplexy: a review of clinical presentation, management and outcome in 45 cases. *Pituitary,* Vol.7, No.3, (March, 2011), pp. 157-163, ISSN 1386-341X.

Semple, P.L.; Webb, M.K.; de Villiers, J.C. & Laws, E.R.Jr. (2005). Pituitary apoplexy. *Neurosurgery,* Vol.56, No.1,(May, 2011), pp. 65-72, ISSN 0148-396X.

Krull, I.; Christ, E.; Kamm, C.P.; Ganter, C. & Sahli, R. (2010). Hyponatremia associated coma due to pituitary apoplexy in early pregnancy: a case report. *Gynecol Endocrinol,* Vol.26, No.3, (May, 2011), pp. 197-200, ISSN 0951-3590.

Lubina, A.; Olchovsky, D.; Brezin, M.; Ram, Z.; Hadani, M. & Shimon, I. (2005). Management of pituitary apoplexy: clinical experience with 40 patients. *Acta Neurochir (Wien),* Vol.147, No.2, (May, 2011), pp. 151-157, ISSN 0001-6268.

Atmaca, H.; Tanriverdi, F.; Gokce, C.; Unluhizarci. K. & Kelestimur, F. (2007). Posterior pituitary function in Sheehan's syndrome. *Eur J Endocrinol*, Vol.156, No.5, (May, 2011), pp. 563-567, ISSN0804-4643.

Iwasaki, Y.; Oiso, Y.; Yamauchi, K.; Takatsuki, K.; Kondo, K.; Hasegawa, H.; Itatsu, T.; Niinomi, M.; Tomita, A. (1989). Neurohypophyseal function in postpartum hypopituitarism: impaired plasma vasopressin response to osmotic stimuli. *J Clin Endocrinol Metab*, Vol. 68, No.3, (June, 2011), pp:560-565, ISSN 0021-972X.

Briet, J.W. (1998). Diabetes insipidus, Sheehan's syndrome and pregnancy. *Eur J Obstet Gynecol Reprod Biol*, Vol.77, No.2, (April, 2011), pp. 201-203, ISSN 0301-2115.

Mehdi, A.A.; Salti, I. & Uthman, I. (2011). Antiphospholipid syndrome: endocrinologic manifestations and organ involvement. *Semin Thromb Hemost*, Vol.37, No.1, (April, 2011), pp. 49-57, ISSN 0094-6176.

Wiser, A.; Hershko-Klement, A.; Fishman, A.; Nachasch, N. & Fejgin, M. (2008). Gestational diabetes insipidus and intrauterine fetal death of monochorionic twins. *J Perinatol*, Vol.28, No.10, (April, 2011), pp. 712-714, ISSN 0743-8346.

Weinberg, L.E.; Dinsmoor, J.E.; Silver, R.K. (2010). Severe hydramnios and preterm delivery in association with transient maternal diabetes insipidus. *Obstet Gynecol* Vol.116, No.(Suppl.2), (May, 2011), pp: 547-549, ISSN 0029-7844.

Nyul, Z.; Vajda, Z.; Vida, G.; Sulyok, E.; Frokiaer, J. & Nielsen, S. (2002). Urinary aquaporin-2 excretion in preterm and full-term neonates. *Biol Neonate*, Vol.82, No.1, (2, 2011), pp. 17-21, ISSN 0006-3126.

Zelenina, M.; Li, Y.H.; Glorieux, I.; Arnaud, C.; Cristini. C.; Decramer, S.; Aperia, A. & Casper, C. (2006). Urinary aquaporin-2 excretion during early human development. *Pediatr Nephrol*, Vol.21, No.7, (June, 2011), pp. 947-952, ISSN 0931-041X.

Iacobelli, S.; Addabbo, F.; Bonsante, F.; Procino, G.; Tamma, G.; Acito, A.; Esposito, L.; Svelto, M. & Valenti, G. (2006). Aquaporin-2 excretion and renal function during the 1st week of life in preterm newborn infants. *Nephron Physiol*, Vol.104, No.4, (4, 2011), pp. 121-125, ISSN 1660-2137.

Bianchi, Y. (2010). Idiopathic central diabetes insipidus in a premature newborn successfully treated by sublingual desmopressin. *Swiss Med Wkly*, Vol.140, No.21-22, (April, 2011), pp. 22S-22S, ISSN 1424-7860.

Stapleton, G. & DiGeronimo, R.J. (2000). Persistent central diabetes insipidus presenting in a very low birth weight infant successfully managed with intranasal dDAVP. *J Perinatol*, Vol.20, No.2, (April, 2011), pp. 132-134, ISSN 0743-8346.

Ng, P.C.; Lee, C.H.; Fok, T.F.; Lam, S.T.; Chan, Y.L.; Wong, W.; Cheung, K.L. & Chan, W.K. (1997). Central diabetes insipidus in a newborn with deletion of chromosome 7q. *J Paediatr Child Health*, Vol.33, No.4, (4, 2011), pp. 343-345, ISSN 1034-4810.

Leichtman, L.G.; Wood, B. & Rohn, R. (1994). Anophthalmia, cleft lip/palate, facial anomalies, and CNS anomalies and hypothalamic disorder in a newborn - a midline developmental field defect. *Am J Med Genet*, Vol.50, No.1, (May, 2011), pp.39-41, ISSN 0148-7299.

Ng, S.B.; W.; Buckingham, K.J.; Hannibal, M.C.; McMillin, M.J.; Gildersleeve, H.I.; Beck, A.E.; Tabor, H.K.; Cooper, G.M.; Mefford, H.C.; Lee, C.; Turner, E.H.; Smith, J.D.; Rieder, M.J.; Yoshiura, K.; Matsumoto, N.; Ohta, T.; Niikawa, N.; Nickerson, D.A.; Bamshad, M.J. & Shendure J. (2010). Exome sequencing identifies MLL2 mutations as a cause of Kabuki syndrome. *Nat Genet,* Vol.42, No.9, (May, 2011), pp.790-793, ISSN 1061-4036.

Amr, S.; Heisey, C.; Zhang, M.; Xia, X.J.; Shows, K.H. & Ajlouni, K. (2007). A homozygous mutation in a novel zinc-finger protein, ERIS, is responsible for Wolfram syndrome. *Am J Hum Genet,* Vol.81, (April, 2011), pp. 673-683, ISSN 1061-4036.

Siahanidou, T.; Tsoumas, D.; Kanaka-Gantenbein, C. & Mandyla, H. (2006). Neuroendocrine abnormalities in a neonate with congenital toxoplasmosis. *J Pediatr Endocrinol Metab,* Vol.19, No.11, (April, 2011), pp. 1363-1366, ISSN 0334-018X.

Muller-Scholden, J.; Lehrnbecher, T.; Muller, H.L.; Bensch, J.; Hengen, R.H.; Sörensen, N. & Stockhausen, H.B. (2000). Radical surgery in a neonate with craniopharyngioma - Report of a case. *Pediatr Neurosurg,* Vol.33, No.5, (April, 2011), pp.265-269, ISSN 1016-2291.

Levendoglu-Tugal, O.; Noto, R.; Juster, F.; Brudnicki, A.; Slim, M.; Beneck, D. & Jayabose, S. (1996). Langerhans cell histiocytosis associated with partial DiGeorge syndrome in a newborn. *J Pediatr Hematol Oncol,* Vol.18, No.4, (May, 2011), pp. 401-404, ISSN 1077-4114.

Barakat, A.J.; Pearl, P.L.; Acosta, M.T. & Runkle, B.P. (2004). 22q13 deletion syndrome with central diabetes insipidus: a previously unreported association. *Clin Dysmorphol,* Vol.13, No.3, (April, 2011), pp.191-194, ISSN 0962-8827.

Kozma, C. (2005). Neonatal toxicity and transient neurodevelopmental deficits following prenatal exposure to lithium: Another clinical report and a review of the literature. *Am J Med Genet,* Vol.132A, No.4, (May, 2011), pp. 441-444, ISSN 1552-4825.

Zerbe, RL.; Robertson, GL. (1981). A comparison of plasma vasopressin measurements with a standard indirect test in the differential diagnosis of polyuria. *N Engl J Med,* Vol.305, No.26, (May, 2011), pp.1539-1546, ISSN 0028-4793.

Fjellestad-Paulsen, P.; Hoglund, S.; Lundin, S, & Paulsen, O. (1993). Pharmacokinetics of 1-desamino-8-D-arginine vasopressin after various routes of administration in healthy volunteers. *Clin Endocrinol (Oxf),* Vol.38, (May, 2011), pp. 177-182, ISSN 0300-0664.

Ray, J.G.;. Boskovic, R.; Knie, B.; Hard, M.; Portnoi. G. & Koren, G. (2004). In vitro analysis of human transplacental transport of desmopressin. *Clin Biochem,* Vol.37, No.1, (April, 2011), pp. 10-13, ISSN 0009-9120.

7

A Case of Central Diabetes Insipidus in a Female Patient with Bipolar Disorder, Lithium Consumer Over the Last Years

Emilio González Pablos[1], Cristina Gil-Díez Usandizaga[2], Maite Cañas Cañas[2], Rosa Sanguino Andrés[2] and Luis A. Flores[1]
[1]*Complejo Hospitalario San Luis. Palencia*
[2]*Complejo Asistencial de Palencia. SACYL. Palencia*
Spain

1. Introduction

Cade described the effects of lithium on manic episodes in 1949. Schou confirmed these initial observations in 1954. From 1949 until today we can speak of the history of psychopharmacology, in fact it is the oldest drug in mental disorders that is still in full use (Johson, 2006).

The Food and Drug Administration (FDA) approved it in 1970 for the treatment of acute mania and in 1974 for the prophylaxis of bipolar disorder.

Today lithium valid indications remain in force: acute mania, bipolar depression, prophylaxis and maintenance of bipolar disorder and unipolar depression. Moreover, its use has also been extended to many diseases: personality disorders, aggression, anxiety, etc. (Freeman, 2006).

However, it is a drug whose management requires detailed knowledge of their numerous side effects (Table 1), as well as drug interactions (Table 2), contraindications and special situations (Álvarez, 2000). The fact that it is a drug with a very narrow therapeutic window, requires frequent monitoring plasma determinations.

We report a case that has, in principle, one of the most common side effects of using this drug, 25 to 35 percent of patients have polyuria and polydipsia (Sadock, 2004), a person who concurrently also presents serious illnesses which require special surveillance. But a close examination proved to be another slightly different pathology documented.

Central diabetes insipidus (CDI) is a condition characterized by polyuria, polydipsia, and nocturia and is due to deficiency of arginine vasopressin (AVP).

The case has already been published four years ago in a Spanish journal (Gil-Díez, 2007), but we consider it of interest in order to report on the progress of the disease and a bibliographic update.

2. Case report

A 61 year old woman diagnosed with bipolar disorder since the age of 18. She was frequently hospitalized due to depressive episodes and treated with lithium for about 19 years with excellent results.

Cardiovascular system	Sinus Node dysfunction ECG changes Myocardial disorders (myocarditis)
Kidney	On Glomerular Filtration Rate (GFR) On Serum Creatinine On Distal Tubular function Renal Tubular acidosis Proteinuria Morphologic changes
Body weight	Increase
Nervous System	Acute toxicity Permanent cognitive impairment Cognitive functions altered
Haematology	Leukocytosis
Skin & Skin appendages	Skin Rash Psoriasis Acne Alopecia
Endocrinous System	Hypothyroidism Increased Calcium plasma levels Glycemic disorders
Gastrointestinal System	Diarrhea Vomiting Constipation Metalic taste
Sexual function	Sexual dysfunction

Table 1. Main Lithium side effects.

Family history: A mother and a brother diagnosed with affective disorder who died by suicide.

Significant medical history and treatment with various specialists: Primary autoimmune hypothyroidism with an adequate replacement therapy treatment, Diabetes mellitus type 2 with current good metabolic control, hypercholesterolemia and obesity.

She was continuously treated with lithium 600 mg three times a day, with appropriate lithemia plasma levels.

Concomitant treatment: Risperidone 3 (0 – 0 - 1/2), Quetiapine 200 (0 - 0 - 1), Levothyroxine 100 (1 before breakfast), Glycazide 30 (1/2 – 1/2 – 0) and Symvastatine 40 (1 at bedtime).

In July 2006, she was admitted for severe depressive episode with suicidal ideation and Paroxetine was added to her treatment. A few days later she suffered from fever, stupor, and myoclonus. Among the studies carried out a plasma lithemia of 1.03 mEq/l was highlighted. Psychotropic treatment was discontinued and she was referred to the Internal Medicine Department. Facing the possibility of a meningo-encephalitis, laboratory tests and CT scan were performed. She was treated empirically with acyclovir, ceftriaxone, and ampicillin, which lead to the disappearance of the fever and other satisfactory outcomes. Micrococcus sp was isolated from blood cultures.

Drug	Effect	Risk*
Ansiolitic - alprazolam, clonazepam	 > lithemia due to > oral lithium absortion	 3
Anticonvulsivants - carbamazepine/valproate - lamotrigine/gabapentin	 > lithemia, neurotoxicity risk ¿?	 2 3
Antidepressants - SSRI - Tricyclic - MAOIs	 > lithemia, serotonin sd. Risk ¿? lithemia, > tremor ¿? lithemia, serotonin sd. Risk	 2 2 2
Antipsychotics - Atypical - Classical	 > lithemia ¿?	 2 2
Calcium Channel Blockers - verapamil, diltiazem	 possible synergism	 1
Risk: (1) Interaction risk, use only if necessary, surveillance; (2) potentially hazard, surveillance; (3) safe, mild discomfort		

Table 2. Lithium interactions with other psychotropic drugs

In this context, high blood sodium levels (164 mEq/l), polyuria and polydipsia were presented. The urine had an osmolarity of 369, lower than would correspond to blood osmolarity of 353 mOsm/kg. The values of 24-hour urine cortisol were increased but with normal baseline figures for plasma cortisol. Also presenting: ADH: 2.8 pg/ml, aldosterone: 273 pg/ml, renin: 0.7 ng/ml/h. Abdominal CT is performed to assess adrenal glands and new determinations of urinary cortisol, ACTH and DHEA plasma levels, all within the normal range. It was thought in diabetes insipidus and detailed assessment was made of Nephrology and Endocrinology Services, to confirm whether it was central or nephrogenic diabetes.

The results of analytical determinations carried out are detailed as follows:

Serum chemistries:

- Blood glucose (82 mg/dl.), Urea (38 mg/dl.), Creatinine (0.66 mg/dl.), Uric acid (5.9 mg/dl.), Triglycerides (151 mg/dl.), Cholesterol (265 mg/dl.), HDL-cholesterol (53 mg/dl.), LDL-cholesterol (182 mg/dl.), Electrolytes (BUN, creatinine, Na, K, Cl all within normal range), Calcium (9.2 mg/dl.), Phosphorus (3.6 mg/dl.), transaminases (normal), blood osmolarity (296 mOsm/Kg.), urine osmolarity in 24 hours (197 mOsm/Kg.), diuresis (4500ml.),
- Nugent test: after administration of 1 mg of Dexamethasone, Cortisol levels post-dexametasone 0.63 mcg/dl.
- Thyroid function: thyroxine free (0.75 ng/dl.), TSH (3.75 mIU/l), FSH (14.1 IU/l), LH (3.72 IU/l.)

- Cortisol in urine 24 hours (65 mcg.),
- Estradiol (29 pg/ml.),
- Growth Hormone (baseline: 0.4 ng/ml. - After 15' lower than 0.3 ng/ml.),
- Prolactin (previous baseline values: 9.1 and 5.8 ng/ml.)

The water deprivation test (WDT) is performed followed by desmopressin injection (DDAVP test). Both test results (table 3) were compatible with partial central diabetes insipidus, due to the appearance of urine concentration after a desmopressin injection as shown in the following results:

- Blood osmolarity at 08:30 h: 297 mOsm/kg.; at 11:30 h: 304 mOsm/kg.; at 14:00 h: 300 mosm/kg.
- In urine from 07:30 to 08:30 h: 138 mOsm/Kg.; from 10:30 h to 11:30 h: 197 mOsm/kg.; from 13:30 h to 14:30 h: 154 mOsm/kg.
- At 14:30 h (with an increased urine osmolality less than 30 mOsm/kg, blood osmolarity> 290 and urine> 300), 2 mcg desmopressin was injected subcutaneously.
- Urine osmolality from 14:30 to 15:30 h: 300 mOsm/kg; from 15:30 to 16:30 h: 402 mOsm/kg.; from 16:30 to 17:30: 351; from 17:30 to 18:30: 269 mOsm/kg.
- Osmolality (4 h after desmopressin injecticon): 295 mOsm/kg; ADH: 1.6 pg/ml. Study being compatible with partial central diabetes insipidus presenting partial concentration of the urine after injection of DDAVP.

In addition, there were no changes in kidney function.

		Blood	**Urine**
Osmolality		296 mOsm/Kg	197 mOsm/Kg
Water Deprivation Test			
Osmolarity (mOsm/Kg)at	08:30 h.	297	138
	11:30 h.	304	197
	14:00 h.	300	154
DDVP test (2 mcgr. Dessmopresin injec.)			
Osmolarity (mOsm/Kg) at	15:30 h.		300
	16:30 h.		402
	17:30 h.		351
	18:30 h.	295	269

Table 3. Water Deprivation and Vassopresin tests results

In the WDT (Muller test), urine osmolality is not modified neither in Central Diabetes Insipidus nor in Nephrogenic Diabetes Insipidus.

In DDVP test, urine osmolality is increased > 9% in Central Diabetes Insipidus.

MRI of the brain and pituitary findings: Partially empty sella, small laminar pituitary gland covering the sella's floor, centred pituitary stalk, no abnormalities suggesting a pathology were showed after contrast administration.

The patient medical history was completed with the following diagnosis: Diabetes insipidus. Partially empty sella. Normal pituitary function.

Desmopressin therapy was prescribed 0.1 mg every 8 hours. A few days later, the volume of urine collected in 24 hours was within acceptable range.

Since our first study, four years ago, the patient has continued to balance psychopathologically and no episodes of mental illness were presented. During this time the patient has been treated with lithium and it's lithemia plasma levels have always been within therapeutic range.

Current treatment:

Lithium 400 mg (1-1-1), Clonazepan 2 mg (½ - ½ -1), Escitalopram 15 (1-0 -0), Quetiapine 100 (0-0-1), Desmopressin 0.1 mg (1-1-1), Levothyroxine 100 (1-0-0), Simvastatin 40 mg (0-0-1), Gliclazide 30 mg (½ tablet od -breakfast-).

During this period the patient attended frequent medical controls with analytical testing. In all cases the patient has remained stable. Related to central diabetes insipidus has remained asymptomatic, with mild polyuria and polydipsia and analytical testing within normal range limits. She continued with desmopressin.

However, the patient was admitted twice for a few days because of respiratory failure and moderate pulmonary hypertension. Treatment includes oxygen therapy, tiotropium 18 mcgr (one puff od), budesonide and formoterol fumarate 160/4.5 mcgr (one puff bd) and torasemide 10 mg (od at breakfast).

3. Discussion

Central diabetes insipidus (CDI) is a condition characterized by polyuria and polydipsia due to the presence of inadequate secretion of antidiuretic hormone (ADH) or vasopressin by the neurohypophysis or posterior pituitary; in the absence of ADH polyuria, itoccurs because the patient is unable to concentrate urine.

Any cause damaging or altering the neurohypophyseal system can lead to CDI (Casanueva, 1998). Traumatic brain injury or neurosurgery are the most frequent causes, there are also primary and inherited forms (Table 4). However, it should be noted that in 25% of cases in adults the etiology remains unknown (Catalá, 2007).

In nephrogenic diabetes insipidus (NDI) lithium interferes with the action of ADH at distal tubule and collector level by reducing the sensitivity of adenylate cyclase to vasopressin and consequently interfering with the formation of intracellular cAMP. As some authors describe, 10% of patients with the chronic treatment of lithium may develop NDI (Pérez-Blanco, 2000).

Differential diagnosis of diabetes insipidus is complex and involves analytical testing (Table 5) and hypothalamic-pituitary magnetic resonance imaging (MRI), together with the consideration of history and the exclusion of other causes (hyperglycemia, hypercalcemia, etc.).

Whilst nephrogenic diabetes insipidus is considered as a possible and relatively common effect of lithium, this drug in central diabetes insipidus is rarely involved in its origin.

According to other authors, the lithium can induce a partial CDI (Pérez-Blanco, 2000). We have found few cases documented and the mechanism of action is not known. In all references found the population studies are people with lithium treatment who develop symptoms of diabetes insipidus by the simultaneous presence of other pathologies: trauma (Olson, 2004), aortic stenosis (Hensen, 1997), cavernous sinus thrombosis (Kamijo, 2003). The role of lithium in the regulation of ADH release is discussed due to its participation in osmolarity and its action on osmoreceptors as controllers of ADH release (Gold, 1983).

Genetic or familial: autosomal
- Dominant (mutations of the gene encoding the AVP-neurophysin II)
- Recessive
- Gene mutations inactivating AVP
- X Q28 linked (gene not identified)
- Deletion of chromosome 7q
- Wolfram syndrome (WFS gene mutation, region chromosome 4p16)

Congenital
- Septo-optical dysplasia
- hypogenesis pituitary
- Cranial midline defects
- Holoprosencephaly

Acquired
- Head injury
- Neurosurgery
- Neoplasms

- craniopharyngioma, pituitary adenoma, pinealoma, dysgerminoma, meningioma,
- metastasis (carcinoma of the lung in male and female breast)
- hematologic: lymphoma, leukemia
- granulomas, histiocytosis, Wegener granulomatosis, sarcoidosis
- infections: chronic meningitis, tuberculosis, syphilis, viral encephalitis, toxoplasmosis
- vascular diseases: Sheehan syndrome, internal carotid aneurysm, bypass surgery, hypoxic encephalopathy
- autoimmune: lymphocytic infundibulohipofisitis
- inflammatory: lupus erythematosus, scleroderma
- toxins: Tetrodotoxin, snake venom
- drugs: ethanol, phenytoin, corticosteroids, alpha agonists
- idiopathic

Modified from: Catalá Bouset et al. Guía clínica del diagnóstico y tratamiento de los trastornos de la neurohipófisis. Endocrinol Nutr. 2007;54(1):23-33

Table 4. Etiology of central diabetes insipidus. Modified from Bauset M. (2007)

	Normal	Central Diabetes Insipidus	Nephrogenic Diabetes Insipidus
Plasma Osmolality (mOsm/Kg)	Normal	Increased	Increased
Urine Osmolality (mOsm/Kg)	Normal	Decreased	Decreased
Urine Osmolality (mOsm/Kg) after water deprivation	> 750	< 300	< 300
Urine Osmolality (mOsm/Kg) after AVP	> 750	> 750	< 300
Plasma AVP (pmol/l)	Normal	Decreased or Normal	Normal or Increased
AVP: Vasopressin			

Table 5. Diabetes Insipidus differential diagnoses

In our case it is appropriate to note the existence of viral encephalitis in the appearance of the picture, so it is worth recalling the pathological images of sella and pituitary findings. Anyway, the case illustrates the difficulties of management of some patients with lithium, and the need for a differential diagnosis in the presence of diabetes insipidus (Posner, 1996) The treatment is also completely different. In central diabetes insipidus desmopressin is the drug of choice for treatment. It is a synthetic analogue of vasopressin, which has a potent antidiuretic effect. In our case, over 4 years has been effective, and did not change the serum sodium levels (one of the risks of use) (Catalá, 2007).

4. References

Álvarez, E., Pérez, V., & Pérez, J. (2000). *Clínica de litio: Teoría y práctica.* ISBN 8495035146, Barcelona: Permanyer.

Casanueva Freijo, F. (1995). Enfermedades del sistema hipotálamo-hipofisario. In A. Domarus, P. Farreras Valenti, & C. Rozman (Eds.), *Medicina interna* (13ª ed.). ISBN 848174106X, Madrid: Mosby/Doyma Libros.

Català Bauset, M., Gilsanz Peral, A., Tortosa Henzi, F., Zugasti Murillo, A., Moreno Esteban, B. & et al. (2007). Guía clínica del diagnóstico y tratamiento de los trastornos de la neurohipófisis. *Endocrinología Y Nutrición, 54*(1), 23-33. ISSN 1575-0922

Freeman, M. P., Wiegand, C., & Gelemberg, A. J. (2006). Litio. In A. F. Schatzberg & C. B. Nemeroff (Eds.), *Tratado de psicofarmacología.* (pp. 597-617). ISBN 9788445814260, Barcelona: Masson.

Gil-Díez Usandigaza, C., Cañas Cañas, M., Sanguino Andrés, R. M. & González Pablos, E. (2007). Un caso de diabetes insípida central en una paciente con trastorno bipolar consumidora de litio desde hace años. *Anales de psiquiatría,*Vol. 23, No. 5, pp. (253-255), ISSN 0213-0599

Gold, P. W., Robertson, G. L., Post, R. M., Kaye, W., Ballenger, J., Rubinow, D., & Goodwin, F. K. (1983). The effect of lithium on the osmoregulation of arginine vasopressin secretion. *The Journal of Clinical Endocrinology and Metabolism, 56*(2), 295-9. ISSN 0021-972X

Hensen, J., Seufferlein, T., & Oelkers, W. (1997). Atherosclerosis, aortic stenosis and sudden onset central diabetes insipidus. *Experimental and Clinical Endocrinology & Diabetes : Official Journal, German Society of Endocrinology [And] German Diabetes Association, 105*(4), 227-33. ISSN 0947-7349

Johson, G. (2006). Eutimizantes (I). El descubrimiento de las propiedades antimaníacas de las sales de litio. . In F. López-Muñoz & C. Álamo (Eds.), *Historia de la psicofarmacología* (2006 ed.). (pp. 761-9). ISBN 9788479034580, Madrid: Médica Panamericana.

Kamijo, Y., Soma, K., Hamanaka, S., Nagai, T., & Kurihara, K. (2003). Dural sinus thrombosis with severe hypernatremia developing in a patient on long-term lithium therapy. *Journal of Toxicology. Clinical Toxicology, 41*(4), 359-62. ISSN 0731-3810

Olson, D. M., Meek, L. G., & Lynch, J. R. (2004). Accurate patient history contributes to differentiating diabetes insipidus: A case study. *The Journal of Neuroscience Nursing : Journal of the American Association of Neuroscience Nurses, 36*(4), 228-30. ISSN 0888-0395

Pérez-Blanco, J. (2000). Efectos secundarios I: Sistema cardiovascular, riñón, peso. In A. Álvarez, V. Pérez, & J. Pérez (Eds.), *Clínica de litio: Teoría y práctica.* (pp. 121-36). ISBN 8495035146, Barcelona: Permanyer.

Posner, L., & Mokrzycki, M. H. (1996). Transient central diabetes insipidus in the setting of underlying chronic nephrogenic diabetes insipidus associated with lithium use. *American Journal of Nephrology, 16*(4), 339-43. ISSN 0250-8095

Sadock, B. J., Kaplan, H. I., & Sadock, V. A. (2007). *Kaplan & sadock's synopsis of psychiatry: Behavioral sciences/clinical psychiatry.* ISBN 9780781773270, Philadelphia: Lippincott Williams & Wilkins.

8

Imaging Manifestations and Techniques in Diabetes Insipidus

Nirmal Phulwani, Tulika Pandey,
Jyoti Khatri, Raghu H. Ramakrishnaiah,
Tarun Pandey and Chetan C. Shah
University of Arkansas for Medical Sciences, Little Rock, Arkansas
United States of America

1. Introduction

Diabetes insipidus (DI) is a clinical condition characterized by excretion of large volume of low specific gravity urine (1). Diabetes insipidus can be central in which there is deficient production of arginine vasopressin (AVP) also known as anti-diuretric hormone (ADH) or nephrogenic in which there is end organ resistance to ADH action (1).

2. Classification

Etiological classification of diabetes insipidus is as follows.

1. Central Diabetes Insipidus (CDI)
    - A. Idiopathic
    - B. Familial
    - C. Structural Causes
        - i. Congenital: Septo-optic dysplasia
          Tuber cinereum Hamartoma
        - ii. Traumatic: Iatrogenic, head trauma
        - iii. Inflammatory: Tuberculous Meningitis
          Sarcoidosis
          Wegener's granulomatosis
          Lymphocytic Hypophysitis
        - iv. Neoplastic:
            - a. Pediatric:
              Hypothalamic glioma
              Craniopharyngioma
              Intracranial Germ Cell Tumors
              Teratoma
              Langerhans Histiocytosis
            - b. Adult: Metastasis
2. Psychogenic: Compulsive intake of large amounts of fluid leading to inhibition of normal vasopressin (2).

3. Nephrogenic Diabetes Insipidus (NDI)
   A. Primary
   B. Secondary: Polycystic kidney disease, drug toxicity such as Lithium toxicity, analgesic nephropathy, reflux nephropathy, amyloidosis, acute tubular nephropathy (1)

3. Etiopathogenesis

Central diabetes insipidus is characterized by decreased secretion of ADH that results in polyuria and polydipsia by diminishing the patient's ability to concentrate urine. Diminished or absent ADH can be the result of a defect in one or more sites involving the hypothalamic osmoreceptors, supraoptic or paraventricular nuclei, or the supraopticohypophyseal tract. In contrast, lesions of the posterior pituitary rarely cause permanent diabetes insipidus, because the ADH is produced in the hypothalamus and still can be secreted into the circulation (1, 3).
Psychogenic diabetes insipidus is caused by compulsive intake of large amounts of fluid leading to inhibition of normal vasopressin (2).
Nephrogenic diabetes insipidus is characterized by a decrease in the ability to concentrate the urine due to resistance to ADH action in the kidney. NDI can be observed chronic renal insufficiency, Lithium toxicity, Hypocalcaemia and tubular interstitial disease (1, 4, 5).

4. Relevant anatomy

Sella turcica is a saddle shaped fossa located in the sphenoid bone. It is bounded by the prechiasmal sulcus, tuberculum sella and by the anterior clinoid processes. Sphenoid sinus lies below and anterior to it. The bony margins of sella are best seen with computed tomography (CT scan). The fatty bone marrow of the bones of the sella creates hyperintense T1 signal on magenetic resonance imaging (MRI). Suprasellar cistern is a CSF space located just above the sella and contains vessels forming the circle of Willis. Optic chiasm is located within the center of suprasellar cistern. On lateral aspect, pair of cavernous sinuses exist which contain internal carotid artery along with oculomotor, trochlear and abducent nerves in addition to the first and second divisions of trigeminal nerve (6, 7).
The pituitary gland occupies the sella turcica and consists of two parts called as anterior (adenohypophysis) and posterior (neurohypophysis) pituitary. These lobes are developmentally and functionally different. Anterior pituitary is formed from the evagination of oral ectodermal tissue called Rathke's pouch, which is derived from the nasopharyngeal tissue during the embryonic period. Posterior pituitary is derived from diencephalic neuroectoderm and is connected to the hypothalamus via pituitary stalk. Antidiuretic hormone and vasopressin are formed in the hypothalamus and travel to the posterior pituitary and are stored there. The pars intermedia is located between the anterior and posterior pituitary and is regarded as vestigial (6-8).
Anterior pituitary constitutes the 75% of entire pituitary volume and occupies the anterior portion of sella turcica. Posterior pituitary occupies the central portion of sella turcica and is surrounded on both sides by two wings of anterior lobe. MRI easily distinguishes both anterior and posterior pituitary lobe. Posterior pituitary often manifests as markedly hyperintense on T1 weighted images and moderately hyperintense on T2 weighted imaging due to the presence of arginine-vasopressin in neurohypophysis. Entire pituitary gland shows contrast enhancement (figure 1) on both CT and MRI (6-8).

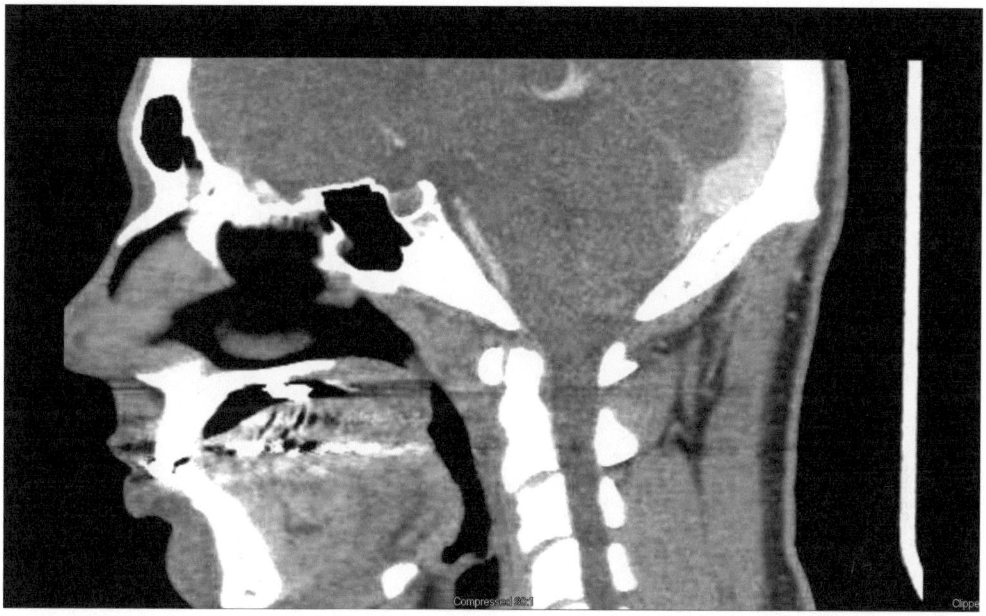

(a)

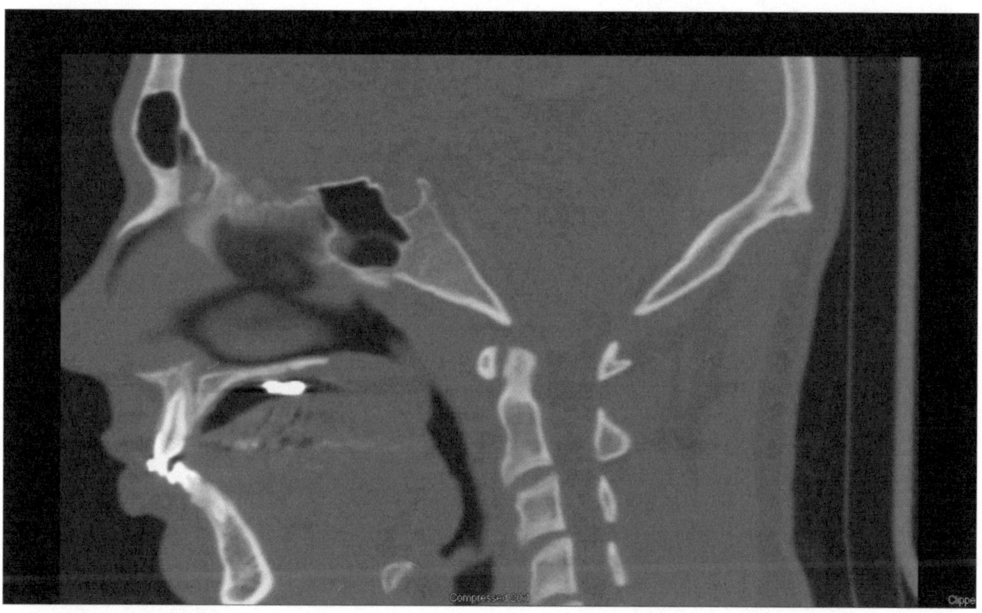

(b)

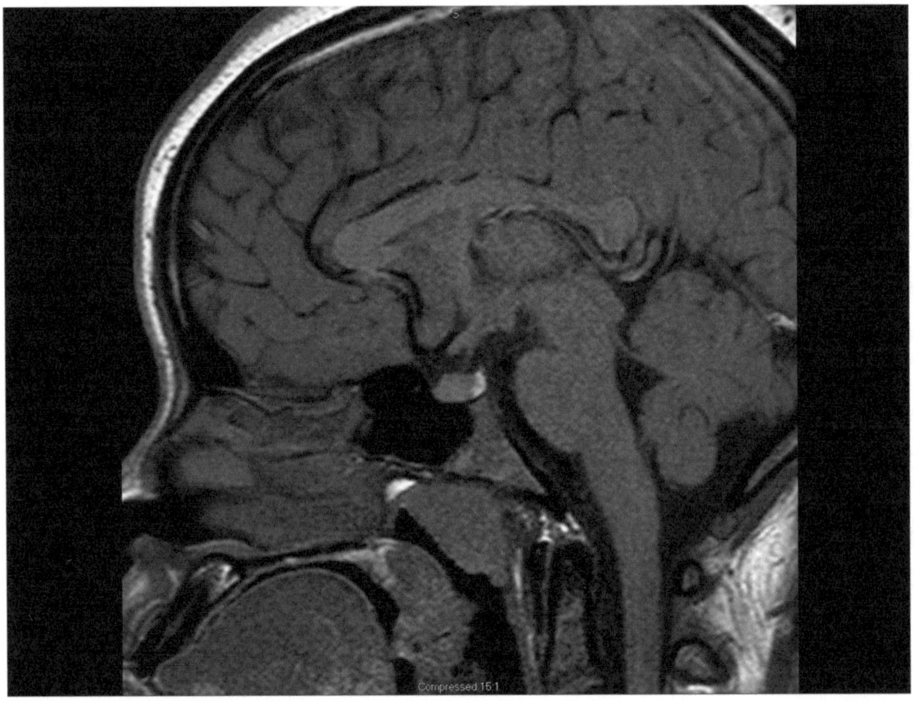

(c)

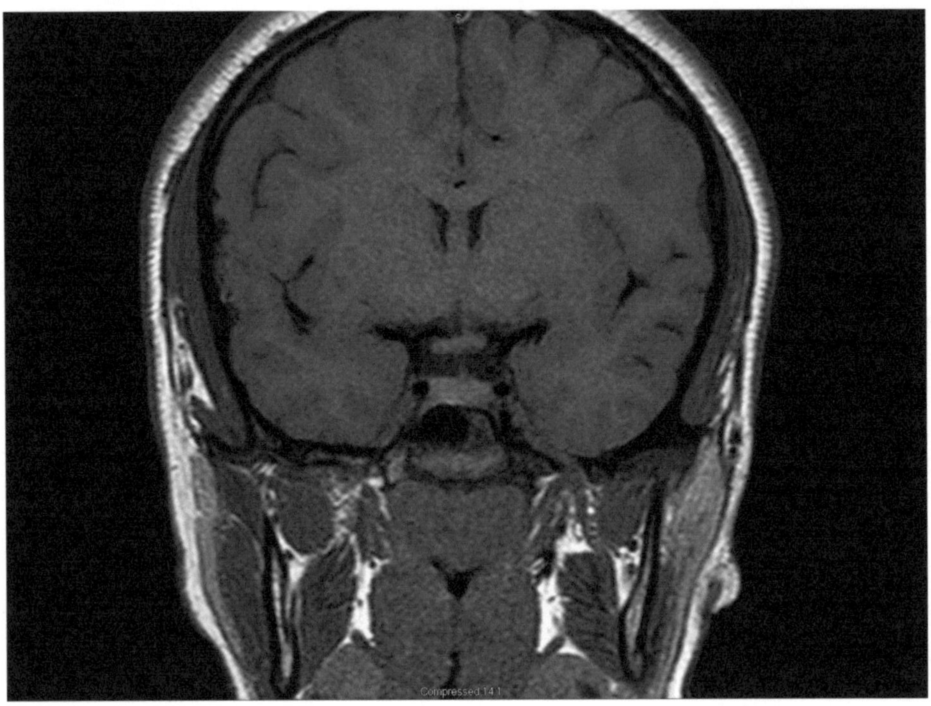

(d)

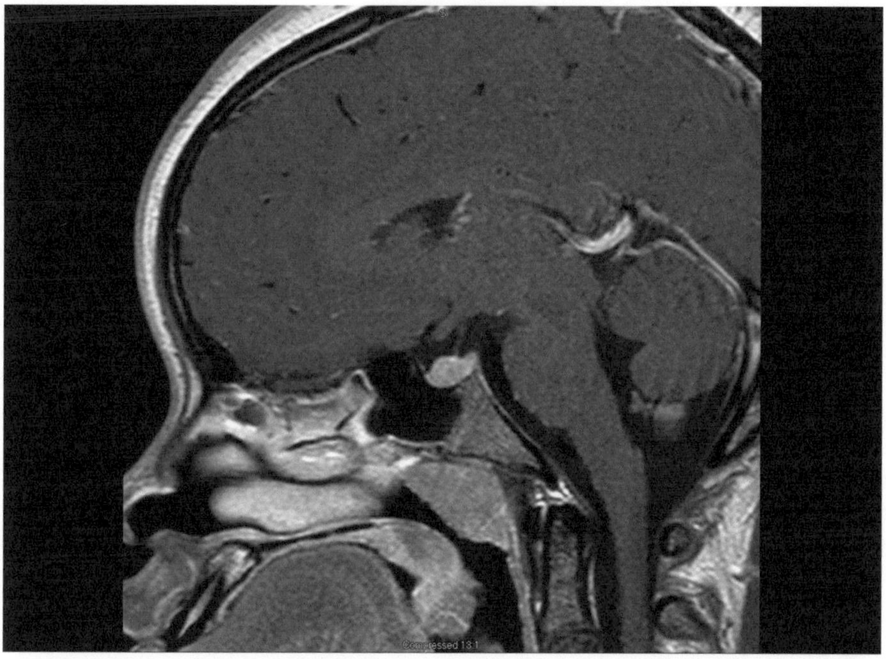

(e)

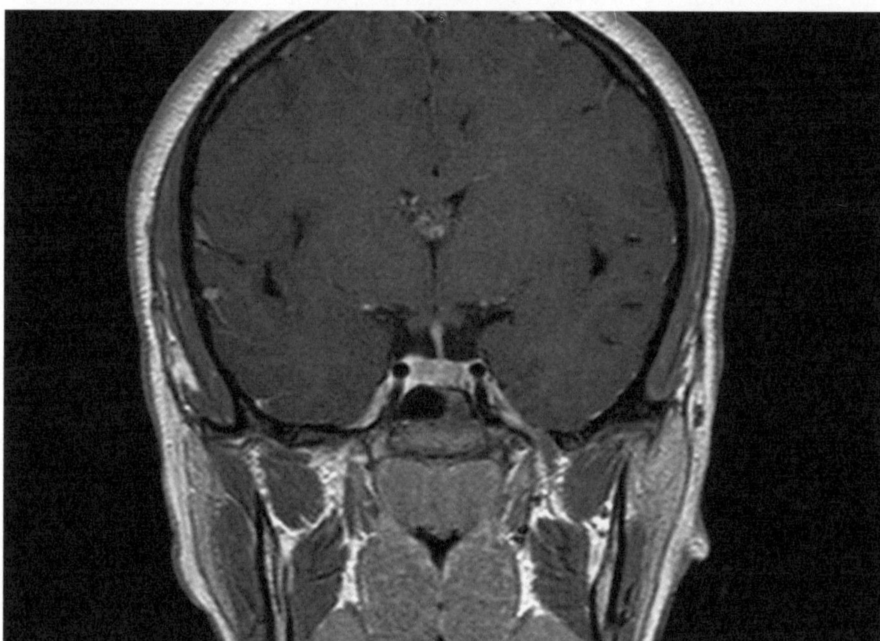

(f)

Normal precontrast sagittal(1c), coronal (1d), post contrast sagittal (1e) and coronal (1f) MRI of pituitary stalk and pituitary gland

Fig. 1. Normal CT sagittal post contrast soft tissue window (1a) and bone algorithm (1b)

The hypothalamus is the ventral part of diencephalon and extends from lamina terminalis to a vertical plane posterior to the mamillary bodies and from hypothalamic sulcus to the pial surface of the floor of the third ventricle (5-6).
Posterior lobe of the pituitary has rich and direct blood supply which explains extensive immediate contrast enhancement of posterior lobe. Anterior pituitary is supplied by the portal pituitary system which explains delay in contrast accumulation in anterior pituitary lobe compared to the posterior pituitary lobe. Similarly, due to relatively deficient vascular supply of anterior lobe, it is more vulnerable to ischemic insults such as Sheehan's syndrome and pituitary apoplexy (6).
Dimensions and shape of pituitary are variable during different physiological states. At birth, pituitary is usually globular in shape and reveals hyperintensity on T1 weighted images in both anterior and posterior lobe. At about 6 weeks of postnatal life, anterior lobe loses hyperintensity and become isointense to that of cerebral white matter. On the other hand, posterior pituitary retains its hyperintensity which serves as an important landmark throughout the life. Pituitary is usually larger in size in female and further increases during pregnancy. Also at adolescent, pituitary size increases physiologically. Despite variations in size, shape and height, pituitary gland should fill the whole sella turcica with variations in height (6-8).

5. Role of imaging

MR imaging is the modality of choice for evaluating central diabetes insipidus due to its multiplanar imaging capability, better tissue contrast resolution and capability to selectively suppress individual tissue signal like fat. CT scan is better than MRI for detecting calcifications, bone destruction and osteolytic lesions (6-8).

5.1 MR imaging protocol

Coronal T1, coronal T2, small field of view sagittal T1 weighted images of the sella with and without fat saturation are obtained., After injection of the intravenous contrast, fat suppressed sagittal and coronal T1 weighted images of the sella are also obtained. MRI of the brain with and without contrast is also performed for a comprehensive evaluation of the pituitary, sellar and parasellar region (6).
Nephrogenic diabetes insipidus is characterized by a decrease in the ability to concentrate urine due to resistance to ADH action in the kidney. Diagnosis of NDI is often clinical and laboratory based and imaging has marginal benefit in this group of DI (1, 4, 5).

6. Central Diabetes Insipidus (CDI)

6.1 Idiopathic Central Diabetes Insipidus

It is the most common type of diabetes insipidus (DI) and is seen in 30-50 % of patients diagnosed with CDI. It has been suggested that idiopathic CDI is an autoimmune disease characterized by the lymphocytic infiltration of posterior pituitary and pituitary stalk. The role of autoimmunity is evident from the association of this disease with other autoimmune conditions and presence of cytoplasmic antibodies against the vasopressin. On MRI, posterior pituitary and pituitary stalk often appear thickened and enlarged, particularly during the early stage. Such presentation is more common in young female patients. However, thickening of pituitary is a non specific finding since patient having such presentation on the MRI, may develop germinoma or histiocytosis. Particularly, progressive thickening of pituitary stalk in pediatric patients on serial MRIs is often due to germinoma. In addition, other endocrine abnormalities are also seen in such patients including suppressed release of growth hormone (GH), thyroid stimulating hormone (TSH) and adrenocorticotropic hormone (ACTH) (3).

6.2 Familial Central Diabetes Insipidus

Familial CDI or familial neurohypophyseal diabetes insipidus (FNDI) is often an autosomal dominant disease which is caused by mutations in the arginine-vasopressin gene (AVP). This mutation leads to accumulation of misfolded arginine-vasopressin fibrillar aggregates within the endoplasmic reticulum and causes death of the magnocellular neurons of SOP and PVN nuclei of hypothalamus. This phenomenon is called toxic gain of function and is also seen in other neurodegerative conditions such as Huntington disease and Parkinson disease. However, it is unclear how these aggregates cause death of magnocellular neurons. Children born with autosomal dominant disease often develop symptoms several months or years following the birth (9).

6.3 Structural causes

6.3.1 Congenital

Septo-optic Dysplasia:

Septo-optic Dysplasia (figure 2) is a disease spectrum with variable combination of the following components:

- Optic nerve hypoplasia
- Pituitary abnormality such as ectopic posterior pituitary
- Absent septum pellucidum

Septo-optic dysplasia is associated with abnormalities of cortical development and hypothalamic-pituitary dysfunction. Suppression of hypothalamic-pituitary axis leads to growth retardation secondary to suppressed release of growth hormone and TSH from the anterior pituitary. In addition, such involvement also affect serum level of ADH since ADH is released from the hypothalamus and stored in posterior pituitary before release into the circulation causing CDI. In addition, these children exhibit variable combinations of cleft palate, syndactyly, ear deformities, hypertelorism, optic atrophy, micropenis, and anosmia (10).

Affected children have mutations in the HESX1 gene, which is involved in early development of the ventral prosencephalon. Pituitary dysfunction leads to diabetes insipidus, GH deficiency and short stature, and, occasionally, TSH deficiency (11).

Posterior pituitary stores hormones released from the hypothalamic neurons which reach posterior pituitary via descending axons. These axons are covered by the ascending ectodermal cells of the Rathke's pouch as they migrate towards the posterior pituitary during development. The development of posterior pituitary is complete by the end of first trimester. Abnormality of the migration can lead to ectopic posterior pituitary gland located either near the median eminence or along the pituitary stalk (12).

Tuber Cinereum Hamartoma

Tuber Cinerium Hamartoma is a congenital disorder of defective neuronal migration characterized by gray matter heterotopias, formation of which typically begins during the

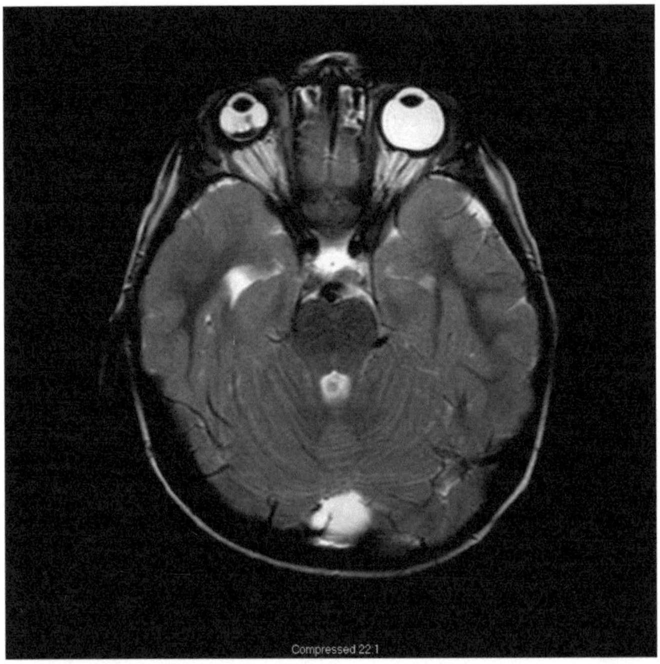

(a)

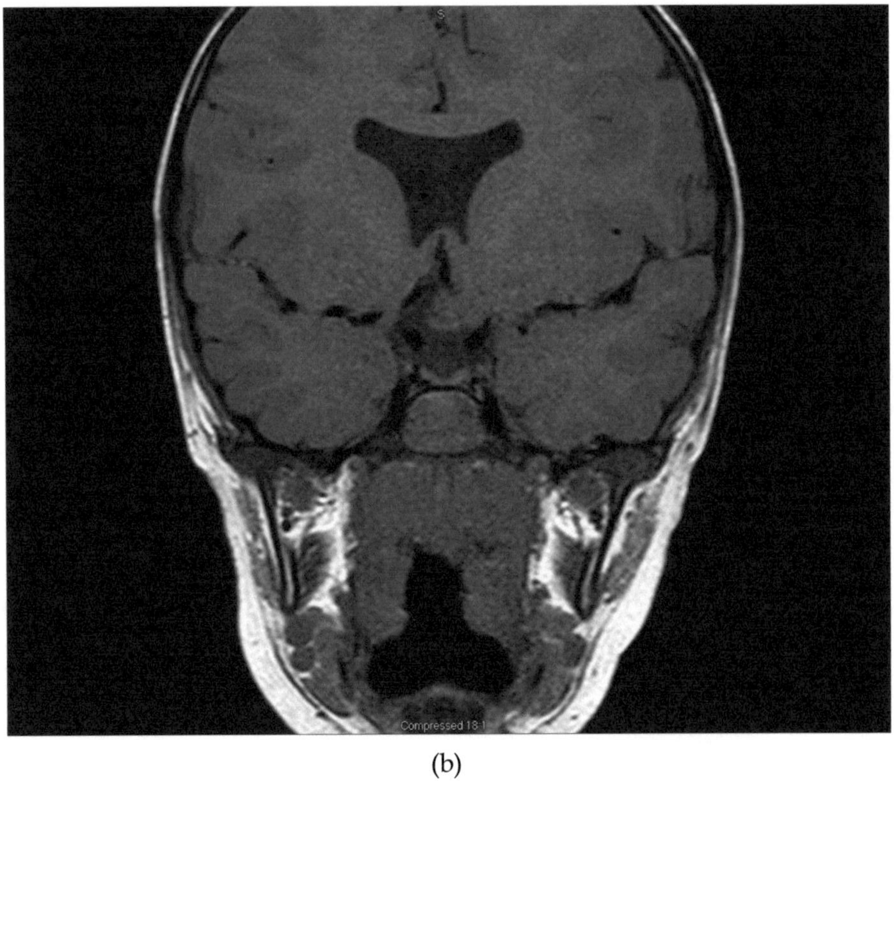

(b)

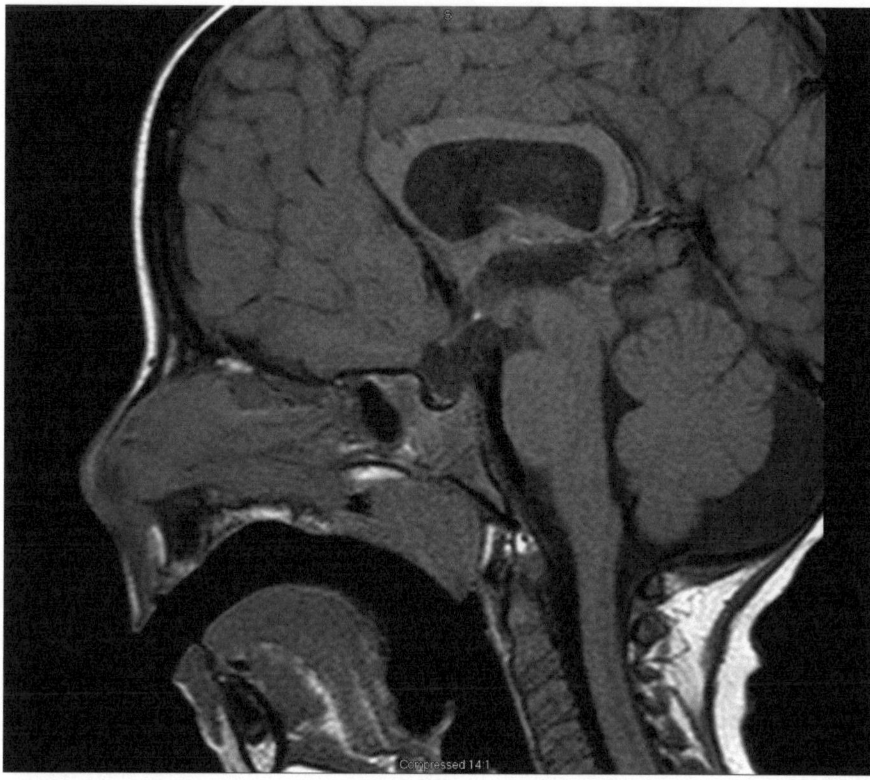

(c)

Fig. 2. MRI of Septo-Optic Dysplasia: Axial T2 (2a) shows bilateral optic nerve hypoplasia, right retinal detachment and right microophthalmia from retinopathy of prematurity. Coronal T1 (2b) shows absent septum pellucidum. Sagittal T1(2C) shows ectopic posterior pituitary bright spot.

days 33-41 of gestational life. It is approximately 1-3 cm in size, nonneoplastic and disorganized collection of hypothalamic neurons, glia and fiber bundles. It is typically located on the floor of third ventricle within the tuber cinereum of the hypothalamus. Recent literature suggested that tuber cinereum hamartoma accounts for about 33% of all cases of true precocious puberty and is seen more commonly in boys than girls. The precocious puberty seen in these patients develops about 2 years earlier than in idiopathic precocious puberty and patients are often less than 3 years of age (13-14).

The induction of precocious puberty is due to pulsatile release of GnRH from the hamartoma which leads to premature activation of hypothalamic-pituitary-gonadal axis. Occasionally patients present with acromegaly secondary to excessive growth hormone release from the Hamartoma. In addition to hormonal disturbances, patient often present with gelastic epilepsy (spasmodic or hysterical laughter) with interval irritability and depressed mood. In addition, several other malformations are also noted in association with tuber cinereum Hamartoma such as polydactyly, microgyria, hemispheric heterotopias, corpus callosum agenesis, mental retardation and behavioral problems. Occasionally, tuber cinereum hemartomas can be a part of Pallister-Hall syndrome which is caused because of a frameshift mutation of chromosome 7p13 and is characterized by multiple malformations, such as polydactyly and imperforate anus. However, neurologic symptoms are less severe in patients with Pallister-Hall syndrome (13-14).

With smaller (3-15 mm) pedunculated mass, patient is often asymptomatic or may only have central precocious puberty. However, with large (10-38 mm) and sessile lesions, patient often display multiple symptoms including seizures. Radiography in patients with tuber cinereum hamartoma and precocious puberty show advanced bone age, evidence of intracranial calcification, increased intracranial pressure and enlarged sella turcica. In addition, ultrasonography shows enlargement of ovaries accompanied by several small cysts/follicles, prominence/enlargement of uterus and well defined central endometrial lining. CT has limited role due to decreased sensitivity at the level of sella turcica and shows isodense mass compared to the gray matter without any evidence of calcification and contrast enhancement. Therefore, MRI is the main modality for identifying hypothalamic hamartoma (figure 3) which shows isodense lesion to gray matter on T1 weighted images which do not enhance with contrast along with preservation of pituitary bright spot. On T2 weighted images Hamartoma is either isointense or slightly hyperintense compared to gray matter. Particularly, lack of enhancement helps to differentiate hypothalamic Hamartoma from germ cell tumor, Langerhans cell histiocytosis and hypothalamic glioma which are also seen in the same location and show at least partial uptake of contrast (13-14).

Recently, it has been reported that MR spectroscopy can also play an important role in diagnosis of tuber cinereum hamartoma with more information regarding the functional status of this mass. Since the mass is slow growing and rarely cause mass effect, initial treatment is symptomatic management and includes hormone suppressive therapy with leutenizing hormone antagonist such as leuprolide or continuous administration of GnRH analogs which effectively suppresses premature precocious puberty and seizures. Surgery is reserved for those patients having intractable seizures or rapid growth of mass with no benefit seen with hormone suppressive therapy (13-14).

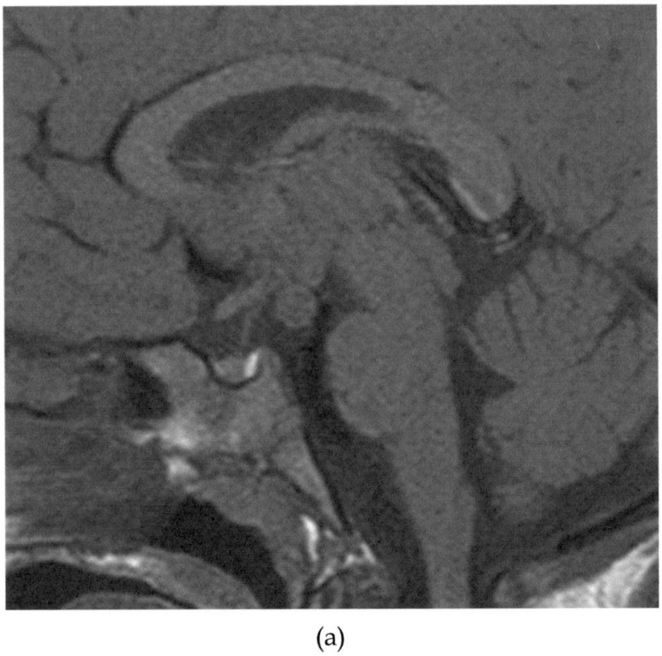

(a)

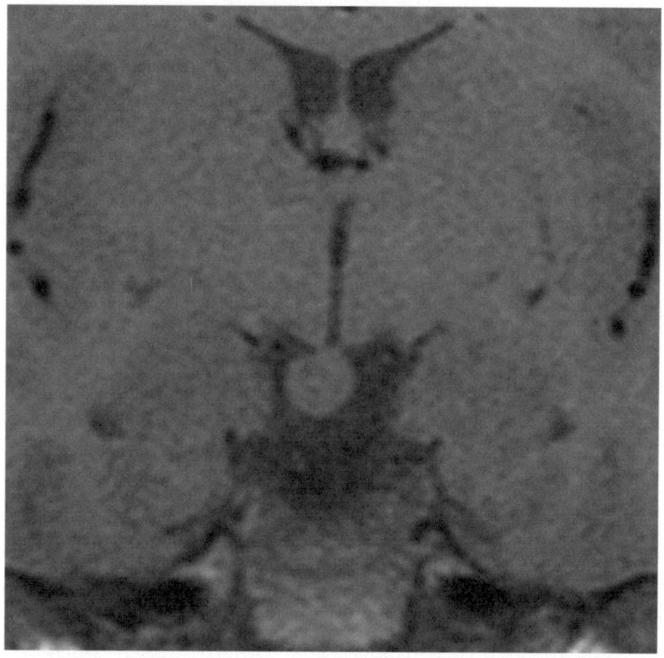

(b)

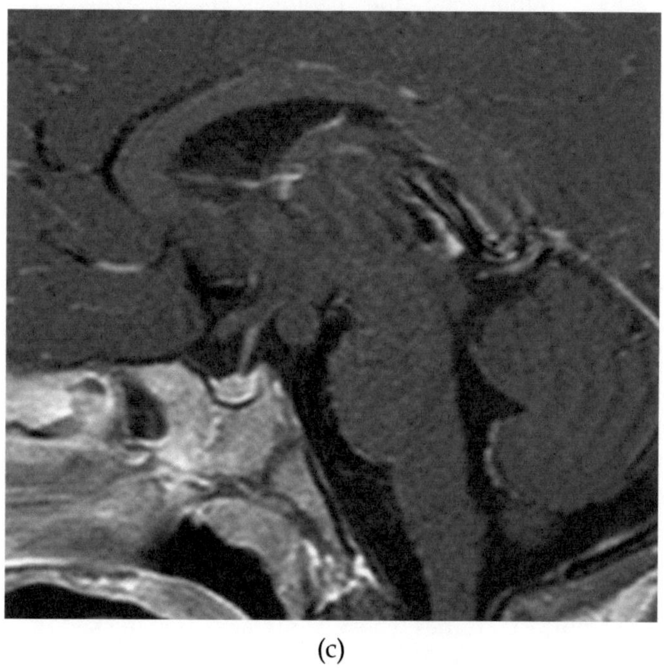

(c)

Fig. 3. Hypothalamic Hamartoma. Precontrast coronal (3a) and sagittal (3b) images show isointense lesion in the region of hypothalamus. Post contrast image (3c) show lack of enhancement of the lesion.

6.3.2 Traumatic

Iatrogenic injury from neurosurgical procedures especially after trans-sphenoidal surgery can lead to the CDI because of iatrogenic damage to the hypothalamus and posterior pituitary. For example, transsphenoidal removal of small tumors limited to sella has resulted in development of CDI. Whereas, removal of large tumors has been shown to precipitate CDI in as high as 60-80% of total patients. The incidence rate declines significantly in patients who have undergone minimally invasive endoscopic pituitary surgery (2.7% permanent and 13.6% transient). The likelihood of developing permanent CDI is higher if plasma sodium level reaches level higher than 145 mmol/L within the first five days postoperatively.

Occasionally, neurosurgery or head trauma causes severe damage to the hypothalamus and pituitary stalk. In such scenarios, often triphasic response is seen. In the beginning, polyuric phase is present which lasts up to 4-5 days and is due to inhibition of ADH release from the hypothalamus. This is followed by antidiuretic phase between days 6-11 that is characterized by the slow release of ADH from the posterior pituitary and leads to hyponatremia secondary to antidiuretic effects of ADH. Once the ADH store in posterior pituitary is depleted, patient develops permanent CDI. However, it is important to note that very often the damage to hypothalamic-pituitary axis is mild to moderate and does not cause permanent CDI. 3.4% of patients had transient polyuria and then transient hyponatremia. It is very important to realize that polyuria seen following a major surgery including neurosurgery is not always due to CDI and may result from excess IV fluids given during the surgery, and also from osmotic dieresis induced from administration of mannitol and glucocorticoid for minimizing the cerebral edema. These conditions can be differentiated from CDI by measuring urine osmolality and the response to water restriction and the administration of ADH. Usually, urine osmolality is less than plasma osmolality and less than 300 mOsm/kg and plasma AVP concentration is low in spite of high plasma osmolality in the CDI Rarely, patient develops combination of CDI and cerebral salt wasting following neurosurgery (15).

6.3.3 Inflammatory

Tuberculous meningitis

Tuberculous meningitis is aseptic meningitis which is often caused because of the spread of infection from the pulmonary focus via hematogeneous route but can also occur because of contiguous spread from adjacent focus of infection. The most common endocrinal disturbance noted is hyperprolactinemia followed by cortisol deficiency and central hypothyroidism. In addition, isolated cases of SIADH and CDI have also been reported.

Intracranial tuberculosis presents as sellar or suprasellar tuberculoma along with calcification, obstructive hydrocephalus, vasculitis or apoplexy. Characteristic MRI changes include sellar tuberculoma, osteomyelitis of adjacent bones, caseous necrosis, dural enhancement and exudates in and around the pituitary gland in addition to thickened pituitary stalk. Post contrast studies show nodularity or thickening of the stalk and infundibulum. The pituitary tuberculomas are heterogeneously isointense on T1 weighted imaging and hyperintense on T2 weighted imaging with intense enhancement with contrast. Occasionally, T1 weighted images show hyperintensity attributed to the high protein content and the non-enhancing areas are likely due to caseous necrosis (16).

Sarcoidosis

Sarcoidosis is a chronic noncaseating granulomatous disease characterized by abnormal collection of chronic inflammatory cells including lymphocytes, macrophages and multinucleated giant cells at various locations including lungs, lymph node, skin and neural tissue. It is more common in African American female. Disease course is often insidious and patient may remain asymptomatic. Occasional spontaneous remissions and improvements have been reported but relapse rate of more than 50% is also seen. About 10% patients develop serious morbidity due to pulmonary scarring and respiratory failure. However, other nonspecific symptoms include fatigue, difficulty to sleep, lack of energy and motivation, joint swelling and pain, blurry vision, skin rash, shortness of breath. Skin lesions include rash, erythema nodosum (swelling in front of anterior tibia or shin) and lupus pernio. There are some variants of sarcoidosis. For example, triad of erythema nodosum, bilateral hilar lymphadenopathy and arthalgia is called Lofgren syndrome that has good prognosis compared to other variants. Involvement of CNS is referred as neurosarcoidosis and is noted in 5% of patients diagnosed with sarcoidosis. In addition, about 33% of patients diagnosed with neurosarcoidosis develop some degree of CDI. In addition, occasional hypothalamic disturbances and defects in anterior pituitary hormonal release are also noted in such patients. Neurosarcoidosis affects leptomeninges, vascular structures, cranial nerves, hypothalamus, infundibular stalk and pituitary gland. DI is suggested to be due to the either vasculitis or direct granulomatous effect.

As with other inflammatory condition involving pituitary stalk, MRI shows uniformly thickened pituitary stalk but occasional involvement of adjacent hypothalamus and pituitary is seen. Similar to other granulomatous disease, strong contrast enhancement is also seen. Interestingly, such features on MRI are seen only in patients who have CDI for less than 2 years and are lost upon follow up suggesting that neurosarcoidosis induced DI is self limiting (17-18).

Wegener's granulomatosis

Wegener s granulomatosis (WG) is a systemic, necrotizing, granulomatous vasculitis of small and medium sized vessels that was first described in detail by Friedrich Wegener in 1939. It is a chronic disease of unknown etiology and is closely associated with elevated serum levels of anti-neutrophil cytoplasmic antibody (ANCA). Once diagnosis is established, WG require lifelong immunosuppresion because of propensity to cause irreversible end organ damage. It affects multiple organ systems, such as upper and lower airway involvement (sinusitis, epistaxis, dyspnea and cough), kidney (impaired kidney functioning, rapidly progressive glomerulonephritis and chronic kidney failure) and other organs. In about one third of patients, CNS is involved and patient exhibit features of peripheral neuropathy, mononeuritis multiplex, cranial nerve palsies, stroke, cerebral vasculitis and rarely CDI. Involvement of posterior pituitary in WG is very rare with only less than 50 cases described in literature so far since 1953. Due to rare association between WG and CDI, it is often missed during the early course of disease. Therefore, it is very important for physicians to suspect WG in any patient presenting with nasal congestion, epistaxis, dyspnea, polydipsia and polyuria. Definitive diagnosis is established by tissue biopsy that often shows leukocytoclastic vasculitis with granulomatous inflammation.

On MRI, WG-induced CDI appear as diffusely enlarged pituitary and infundibular stalk compared to optic chiasm and occasionally intrasellar mass is seen. In addition in some patients, cystic changes have been reported in pituitary and infundibulum but no contrast enhancement is seen. Loss of posterior pituitary bright spot is seen on T1 weighted images (likely due to significant decrease in arginine-vasopressin content in posterior pituitary) and no contrast enhancement is noted. Occasionally, MRI failed to show any changes in pituitary in patients with proven clinical CDI and WG. In such patients, it has been suggested that CDI is caused because of small vessel vasculitis and therefore remain undetected. Treatment is often directed at immune suppression (19-20).

Lymphocytic infundibuloneurohypophysitis and lymphocytic adenohypophysitis

Lymphocytic Infundibuloneurohypophysitis and Lymphocytic Adenohypophysitis were initially identified as one of the most important causes of idiopathic DI. Lymphocytic Adenohypophysitis is a rare autoimmune disease which is seen more commonly in younger female of menstrual age and is acute in onset. Patients often have other autoimmune disease as well and are positive for autoantibodies against arginine-vasopressin secreting cells. It is not yet clear whether these antibodies are cytotoxic and cause DI via damaging the neural tissue. However, their presence indicates the high likelihood of development of overt DI in such patients. Such patients have long history of subclinical disease followed by clinically obvious DI.

MRI in lymphocytic adenohypophysitis typically shows pituitary infundibulum thickening and neurohypophysis enlargement in such patients. During the early subclinical phase, posterior lobe of pituitary is often hyperintense on MRI but become normal again indicating the self-limiting nature of this disease. Upon biopsy, inflammatory infiltrate consisting of T lymphocytes and plasma cells is identified in the affected tissues with occasional presence of macrophages, neutrophils and eosinophils in the anterior pituitary. Interestingly, treatment with DDAVP leads to recovery of posterior pituitary function along with disappearance of autoantibodies.

Lymphocytic Infundibuloneurohypophysitis presents with the combination of CDI and vision disturbances and might have serum positivity for autoantibodies against arginine-vasopressin secreting cells. Lymphoplasmacytic infiltrate is seen in hypothalamus, pituitary, infundibulum, optic nerve, tract and chiasm. MRI imaging in these patients show normal pituitary with focal nodular thickening of the infundibulum, stalk thickening, and absence of hyperintense signal of neurohypophysis. Occasionally, anterior pituitary is also affected. Overall, it is also a self-limiting disorder and no treatment is needed except hormone replacement for short duration of time. In addition, glucocorticoid therapy is also given to decrease the intracranial pressure (21-22).

6.3.4 Neoplastic

6.3.4.1 Pediatric neoplastic causes

Hypothalamic glioma

Hypothalamic gliomas are low-grade tumors arising from glial cells and are classified as World Health Organization grade I tumors. Despite low grade, these tumors are associated with higher morbidity and mortality. Very often these tumors are located in optic chiasmatic/hypothalamic region but are also seen in the posterior fossa, temporal lobe and spinal cord. Hypothalamic gliomas are commonly seen in childhood and adolescent age group. However, hypothalamic gliomas are occasionally seen in adults and are more aggressive than their pediatric counterparts. Male and female are equally affected.

About one third of the hypothalamic gliomas are associated with neurofibromatosis 1, which is an autosomal dominant disease resulting from mutation on chromosome 17. Patients who have associated NF1 have been reported to have better prognosis than those without NF1 and are characterized by smaller, often non-cystic lesions with more frequent involvement of the orbital portion of optic nerve. On the other hand, gliomas without associated NF1 are larger, cystic and frequently affect hypothalamus and optic chiasm. In severe cases, calcification is noted within the stroma of hypothalamic glioma, making it hard to distinguish from craniopharyngioma. Clinical presentation includes headache, visual disturbances, failure to thrive, hyperactivity and endocrinal disturbances such as diabetes insipidus.

On CT scans, hypothalamic gliomas are hypodense compared to the gray matter whereas on MRI, the mass (figure 4) is hypointense to isointense on T1 weighted images and hyperintensive on T2 weighted images. The contrast enhancement is variable but usually mildly homogeneous. Large gliomas may have cystic component that is hypodense on CT and hyperintense on T2 weighted MRI. T2 weighted images are useful for delineating the spread of tumor along the optic tract. Angiography is performed in case of giant and rapidly growing tumors with signs of malignant transformation identifying cerebral vessel displacement and enhancement of abnormal vascular tumor net. Treatment is based on the aggressiveness of the tumor and often involves the combination of surgery, chemotherapy and radiotherapy (23-24).

Craniopharyngioma

Craniopharyngioma (CPH) is a benign tumor, which derives from Rathke's pouch. It is postulated to arise from cells of the embryonic epithelium lining the pharyngeal-pituitary passage extending from the bottom of third ventricle up to the wall of pharynx. It constitutes 10% of all pediatric brain tumors, 90% of all pituitary masses and 56% of all chiasmal-sellar tumors. Two varieties have been identified including cystic (or adamantinomatous) tumors (ACPs) and squamous-papillary variety that are markedly different both clinically and pathologically.

ACP is more commonly seen and is often noted in pediatric patients (between 5-10 years of age). It is characterized by one or more large cysts with variable wall thickness and central proteinacious fluid that has machine oil consistency. In addition, it also has variable proportion of solid component. Overall, it is an inhomogeneous mass commonly associated with both solid and cystic component and some degree of calcification in more than 90% of cases. It is commonly seen in sellar and suprasellar location.

Squamous papillary variant is often solid in nature and rarely present with cystic component. Calcification is not commonly seen. They are often large masses and lead to mass effect and location specific manifestations. Patient often develop Horner syndrome, neurological deficit, epilepsy, headache, pseudotumor cerebri and elevation in intracranial pressure.

It is associated with CDI both before and after the curative surgery with higher incidence noted postoperatively. Interestingly, patients who underwent transfrontal removal of craniopharyngioma have no biologically active ADH in the serum despite elevated level of immunoreactive ADH. In addition, replenishment of ADH level is not effective. This presentation mimics nephrogenic DI. However, CDI in this setting is often transient.

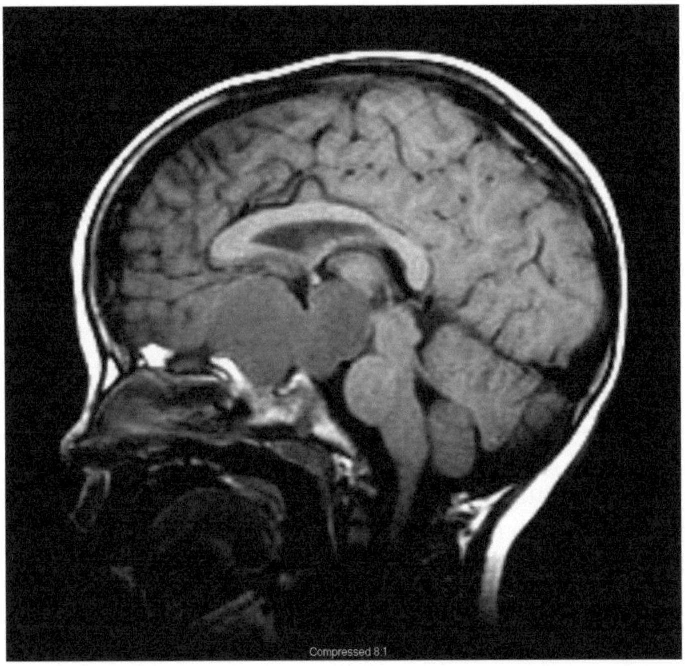

(a)

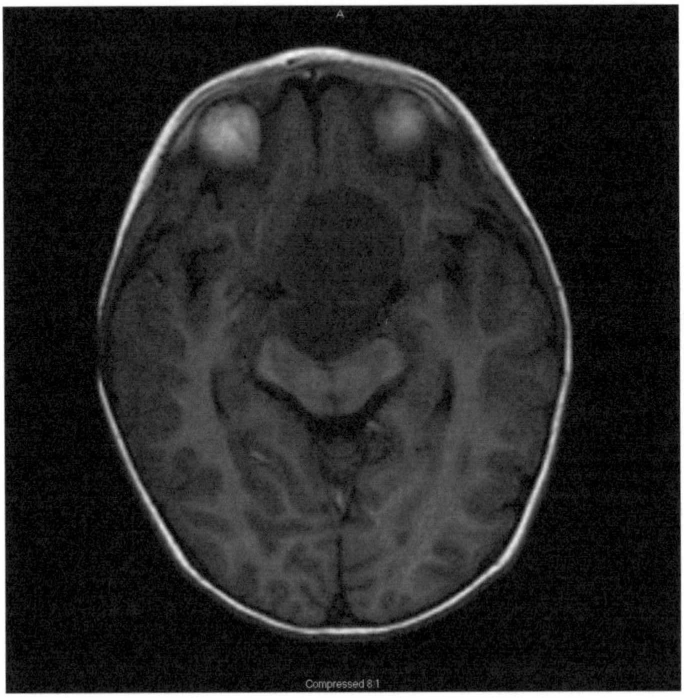

(b)

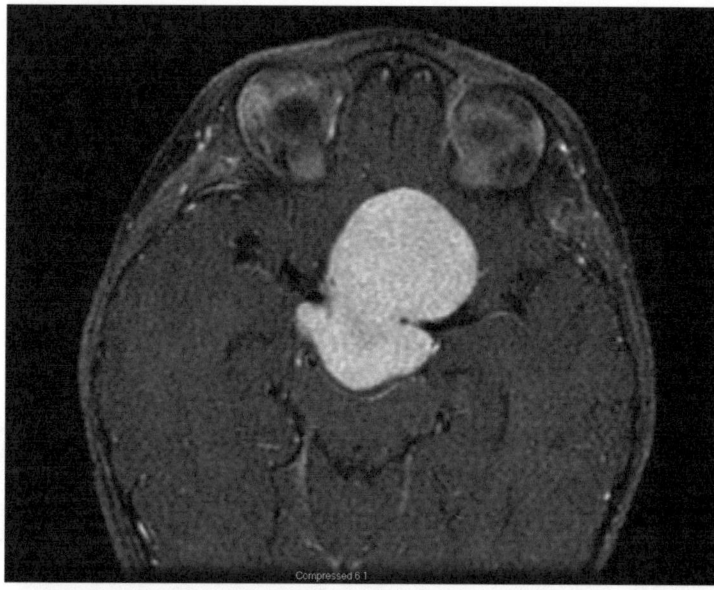

(c)

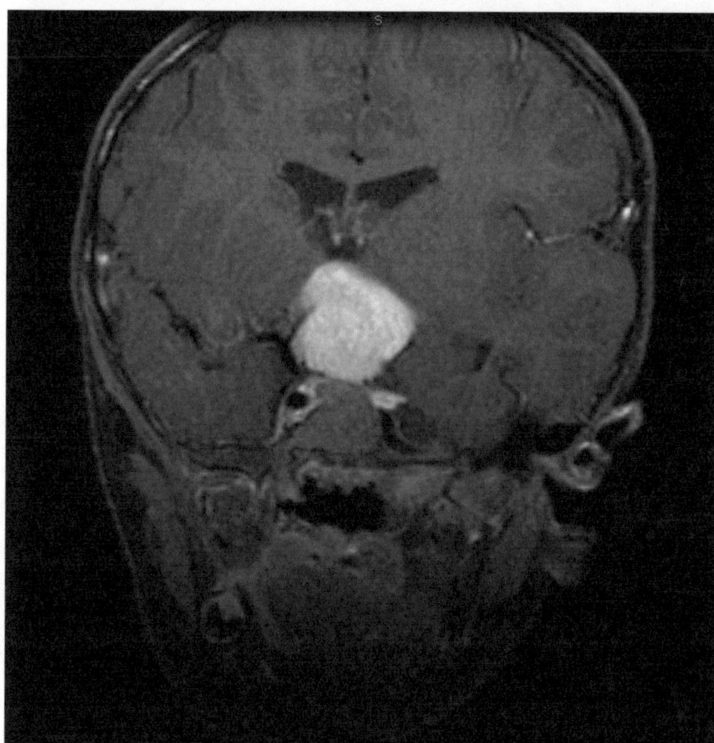

(d)

Fig. 4. Hypothalamic Glioma: Precontrast sagittal T1 (a), axial T1 (b), post contrast axial T1 (c) and coronal T1 (d) images of pilocytic astrocytoma involving hypothalamus

Imaging is very important for identifying CPH, and for delineating the location and extent of craniopharyngioma (figure 5). For example, plain radiography reveals changes in shape and size of the sella turcica, deformity of the anterior clinoid process along with calcifications in the chiasmal-sellar region. In addition, calcification is often seen within the cavity of sella and often present as laminar pattern of calcification within the capsule. In majority of the patients with CPH, the dorsum sella turcica is shortened. Mass effect on the third ventricle causes increase in intra-ventricular pressure with dilatation of ventricular system and widening of bony sutures. CT and MRI provide more detailed and accurate description of CPH, including precise size of the tumor, proportion of solid and cystic component, location, and involvement of ventricular system and erosion into adjacent structures.

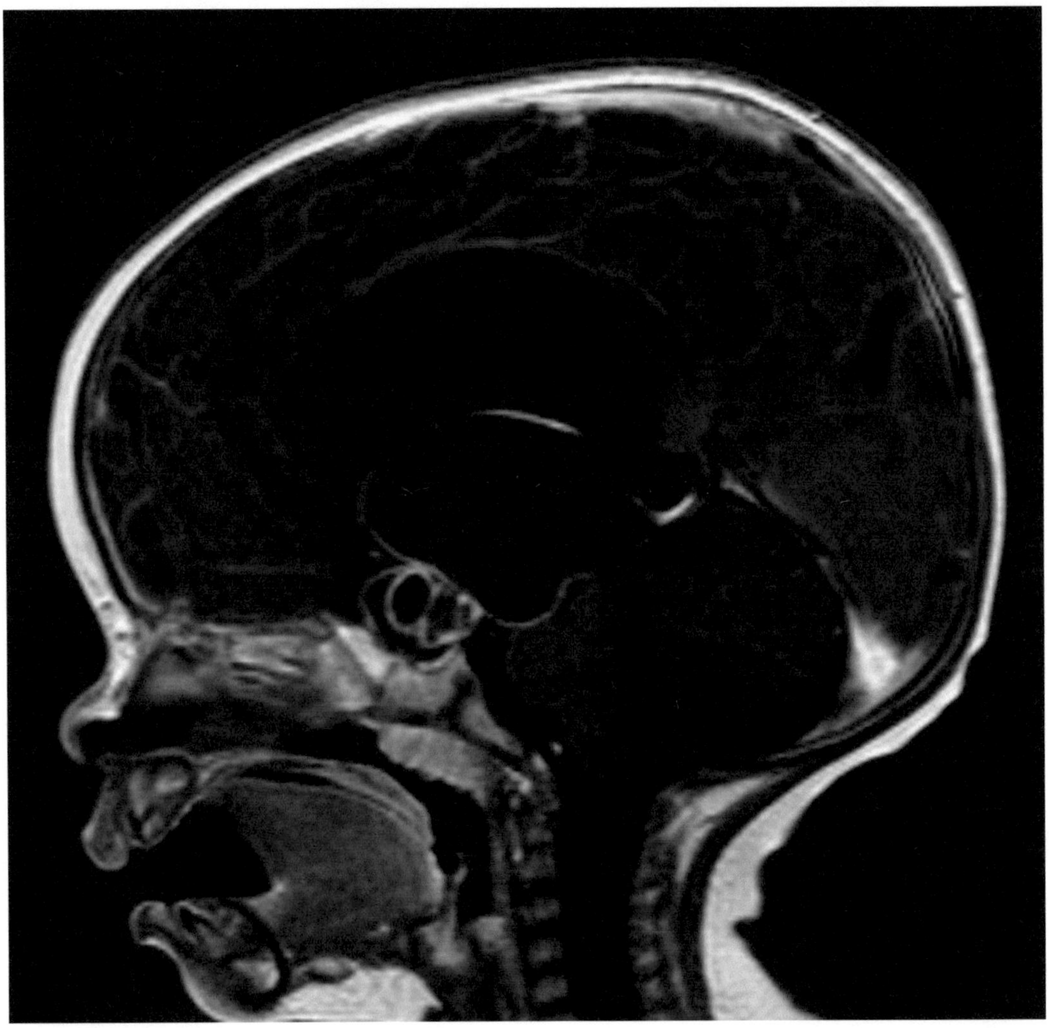

Fig. 5. Sagittal T1W post contrast MR image shows a complex solid and cystic sella-supra sellar enhancing mass. This was a proven Craniopharyngioma on histopathology.

On CT, it appears as a well defined mass with heterogeneous density. Solid part is isodense to the brain but cystic part is usually hypodense than that of brain. Density of solid component increases considerably upon contrast enhancement. CT may show hypodense lesion within the ventricles with peripheral rim of calcification. T1 weighted MR images of cystic component are often heterogeneous ranging from hypointense to hyperintense signal depending on the protein content of cyst whereas the solid or nodular part of tumor is usually isointense. On T2 weighted images, cystic area appears hyperintense with hypointense foci representing calcification. Proteinacious nature of the cystic fluid causes hyperintense signal on T1weighted images and mild hyperintensity on T2-weighted imaging at the periphery. On sagittal images, sedimentation phenomenon of cystic content can be seen. On MRI, intense contrast enhancement is seen in the wall of the cyst and also in the solid component of the tumor (25-26).

Intracranial germ cell tumors

Intracranial germ cell tumors often located close to the midline and could be both benign and malignant. Germ cell tumors arise due to defective migration of primordial germ cells and are commonly seen within the gonads, mediastinum or in the pineal region. In fact more than 50% of tumors within the pineal regional are germ cell tumors. It usually presents between the age of 10-12 years and males are more frequently affected if tumor is located within the pineal regions whereas slight female preponderance is noted in case of suprasellar germ cell tumors. Most of the intracranial germ cell tumors are within the pineal region and 20% are seen in suprasellar region and few are identified in the pituitary fossa. AFP and b-HCG levels are elevated in patients with germ cell tumor and are routinely used for screening purpose and monitoring response to treatment. They constitute 3-5% of pediatric intracranial tumors and 0.5-1% of adult intracranial tumors. Common clinical features are endocrinal disturbances such CDI, precocious puberty and panhypopituitarism. In addition, obstructive hydrocephalus, visual defects and optic nerve atrophy are also seen. On CT, germ cell tumors (figure 6) appear as hyperdense lesions with homogeneous contrast enhancement. It often shows abnormal subtle pituitary stalk thickening and enhancement in patients with CDI. On MRI, germinoma are isointense or mildly hypointense on T1 weighted images and isointense or mildly hyperintense on T2 weighted images. Strong contrast enhancement is seen on both CT and MRI. Treatment of choice is radiotherapy with excellent prognosis. Chemotherapy is used in radiotherapy resistant tumors (27-28).

Teratoma

Teratomas are usually benign tumors which contain elements derived from all the three germ layers and are covered by a capsule. They are commonly seen in pediatric male patients. When located intracranially, these lesions have predilection for the midline and involve the pineal region, the third ventricle, and the infundibulochiasmal region. Rarely, intracranial suprasellar teratomas extend into the pituitary fossa, with enlargement of the sella turcica, thereby resulting in visual disturbance, DI, and hypopituitarism.

Sella is often enlarged with widening of the entry and depression of the bottom. Often teeth like inclusions are seen with in the sella and around it. Occasionally, initial MRI may fail to identify the mass. However, upon follow up with T1- and T2-weighted MR imaging, high signal intensities representing fat components can be seen in sellar and suprasellar areas. Very often, MRI reveals teratomas as heterogeneous mass secondary to the presence of all three germ line structures which enhance following contrast administration (29-30).

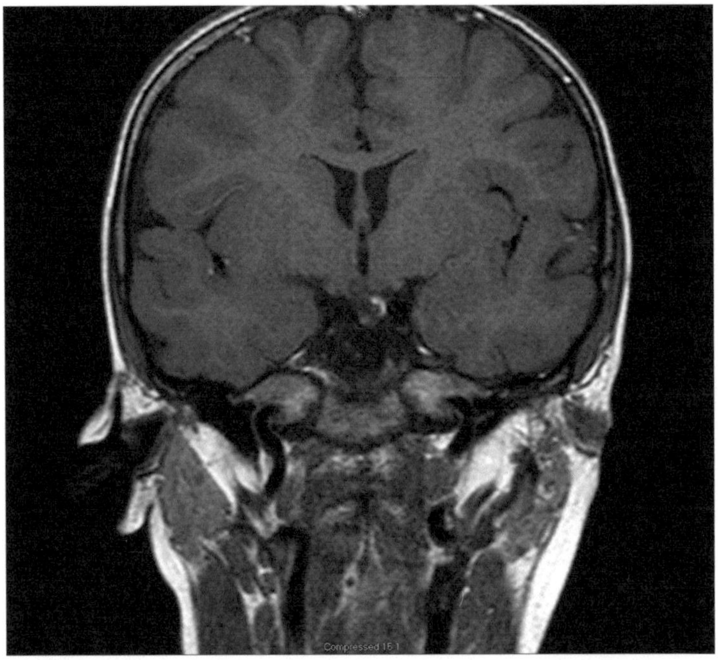

(a)

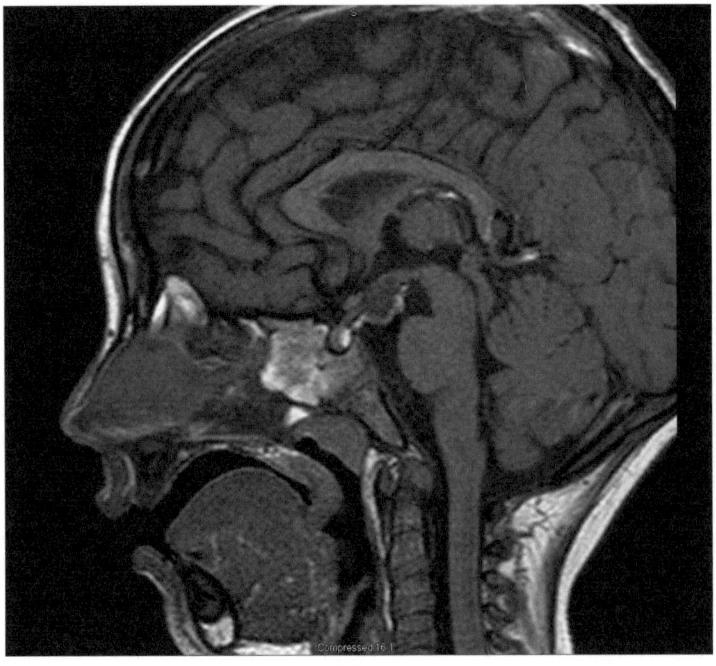

(b)

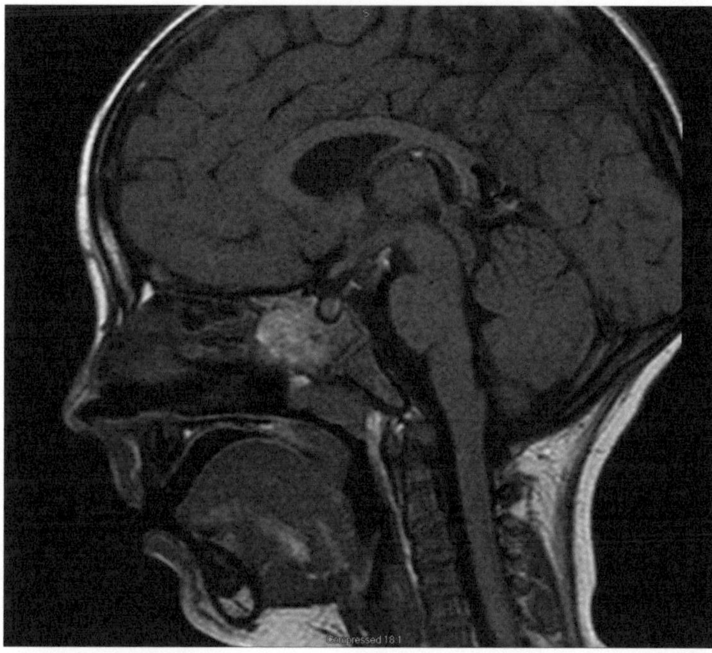

(c)

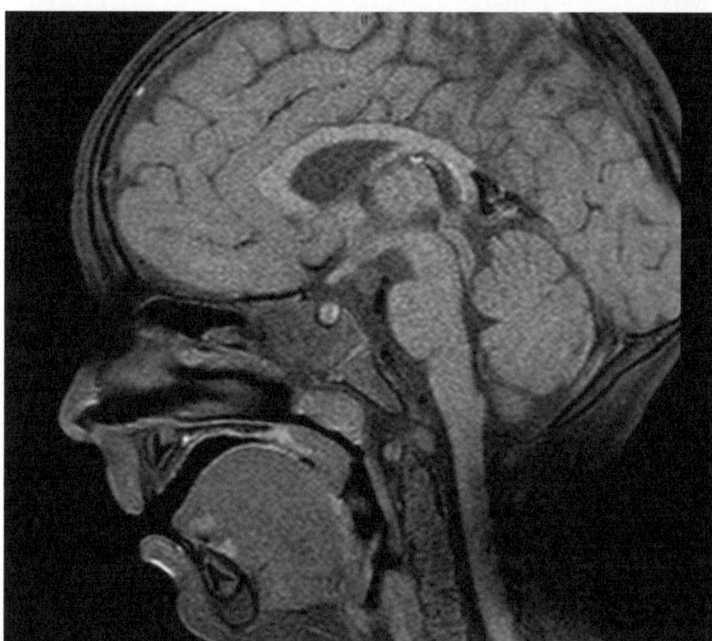

(d)

Fig. 6. Hypothalamic Dermoid: Non-fat suppressed coronal T1 (a) and sagittal T1 (b,c) shows hyperintense T1 signal in the hypothalamic mass that suppresses on fat suppressed T1 sagittal (d) image representing fat in the dermoid.

Langerhans cells histiocytosis

Langerhans Cells Histiocytosis refers to the group of granulomatous disease characterized by abnormal activation and clonal proliferation of immune cells called histiocytes or Langerhans cells and is mostly seen in children between 1-4 years of age. These cells are bone marrow derived and are a variant of dendritic cells that normally reside in the skin. Upon entry of foreign antigen into body via breach of skin, these cells engulf and process these antigens and migrate to the nearby lymph node. They present these antigens to the macrophages and other immune cells and activate the cascades of both cellular and humoral immune response against the foreign antigen. However, upon abnormal activations, these cells can lead to the granumatous disease causing erosive and painful bone lesion in addition to effect on multiple other organ systems.

There are three variants of histiocytosis including malignant (true histiocytic lymphomas), reactive (benign histiocytosis) and Langerhans cell histiocytosis (LCH). Depending upon the nature of bone involvement, LCH is further classified into three variants including unifocal, multifocal unisystem, and multifocal multisystem. In all these variants, LCH provokes nonspecific immune response and leads to painful bone swelling, erosive bone lesion and pathologic fractures, hepatosplenomegaly, lymphadenopathy, pancytopenia, infection, fever, skin rash, hormonal disturbances including diabetes insipidus, chronic cough, shortness of breath and granulomatous lung disease. LCH is commonly seen in pediatric patients and twice common in boys than girls.

Frontal bone is most commonly involved however any bone can be affected and develops punched out lesions with sharp margins and no sclerosis. Particularly, chronic recurrent form is referred as Hand-Schuller-Christian disease which presents as a triad of Diabetes insipidus, proptosis and destructive bone lesions. On the other hand, acute form of disease is called as letterer-siwe disease which presents with hepatomegaly, splenomegaly, fever, eruptive skin lesion, thrombocytopenia and anemia. Diagnosis is established via biopsy and immunohistochemistry with positive reactivity for CD1a and S-100 proteins. In addition, electron microscopy shows abnormal membranous aggregates of endoplasmic reticulum in tennis racket shaped or rod shaped structures called birbeck granules or birbeck bodies (200-400 nm in width). These bodies characteristically show central linear density and a striated appearance and are regarded as pathognomic of histiocytosis. It is reported that formation of these bodies is induced by Langerin (CD207), which is transmembrane II surface receptor present on the membrane of Langerhans cells. Clinically, several hormonal disturbances are seen but the most common is diabetes insipidus followed by growth retardation. In addition, galactorrhea, hypogonadism and hypopituitarism are also occasionally seen secondary to histiocytic infiltration of hypothalamus and partial or complete inhibition of the release of hypothalamic trophic hormones which subsequently suppresses pituitary hormonal release.

On radiographs, variable sized lytic foci are seen with characteristic beveled edge appearance of lesion margin. Occasionally, focal residual bone lesion with button sequestrum is also seen lying centrally within the area of lytic lesion. On CT scan, button sequestrum lesions are seen as sharply defined hypodense intradiploic bony defects. In addition, lytic foci and erosive changes are also seen on CT scans. On MRI, button sequestrum lesion appears as low to intermediate intensity lesion on T1 weighted images and hyperintensity lesion on T2 weighted images. In addition, contrast enhancement with fat suppression enhances the diagnostic yield and helps identify the extent of lesion, invasion of adjacent epidural space, brain parenchyma or dural venous sinuses. In addition, scintigraphy is also helpful but show variable isotope uptake, such as smaller lesions show enhanced uptake and less or no uptake in bigger lesions. This modality help identify multiple osseous and tissue lesions and is of use for narrowing the differential diagnosis. Pituitary MRI (figure 7) will show enhancing thickened pituitary stalk (31-32).

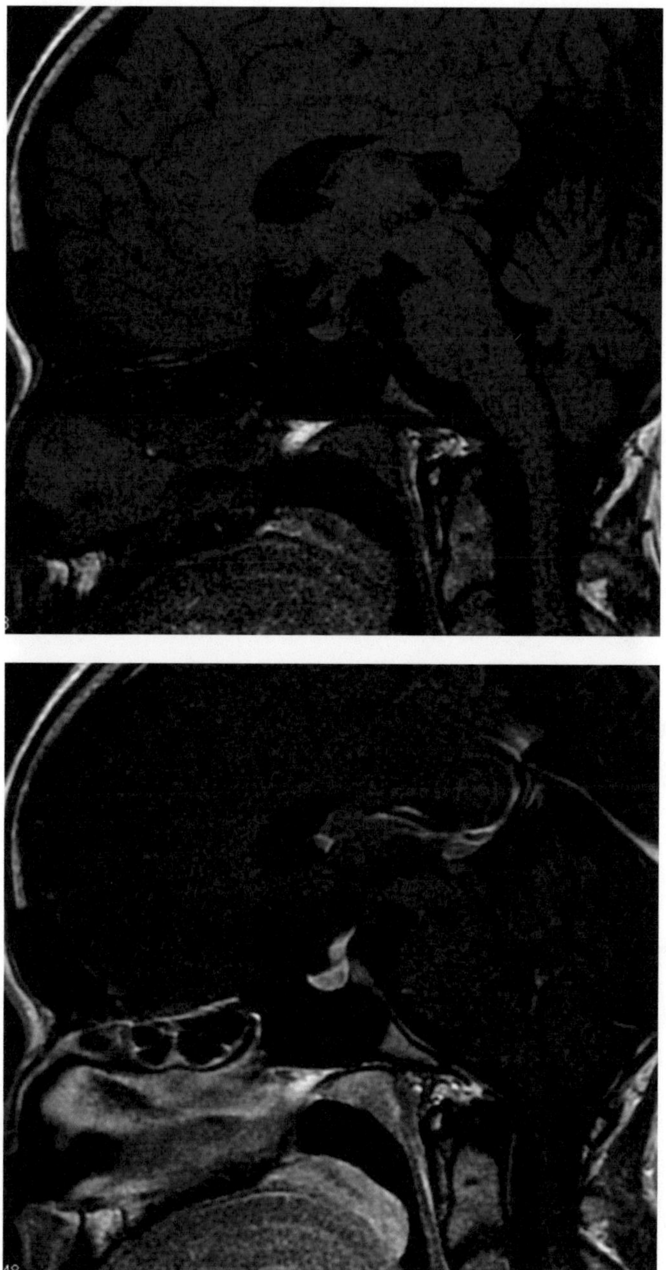

Fig. 7. Histiocytosis involving the pituitary infundibulum. Sagittal non contrast T1W MR image (top) shows absent posterior pituitary bright spot with thickened enhancing pituitary infundibulum on post contrast T1W sagittal MR image (bottom).

6.3.4.2 Adult neoplastic causes

Metastasis

Metastases to the pituitary-hypothalamic axis account for less than 1% of all the sellar masses. Breast cancer metastases are most common, accounting for 6-8% of all the metastasis to the pituitary followed by lung and GI cancers. When cancers metastasize to pituitary, most cancers involve the neurohypophysis but breast cancer demonstrates high affinity for the adenohypophysis. DI is the most common presenting symptoms in such patients and is seen in about 20% of such patients. Other manifestations include vision problems, anterior pituitary dysfunction, headache and ophthalmoplegia. It is permanent if SOP and PVN nuclei of hypothalamus are involved. If SON and PVN nuclei are spared and only posterior lobe of the pituitary is involved, than CDI is often transient.
MRI is very useful for diagnosis and shows a destructive and inhomogeneously enhancing lesion extending across intrasellar and suprasellar location. In addition, diffuse enlargement of the gland, thickening of the pituitary stalk, invasion of the cavernous sinus, and sclerosis of the surrounding sella turcica can also be noted. If metastasis is localized to the skull base, sclerosis of sella turcica is more obvious. On the other hand, if metastasis is located within the pituitary parenchyma, sella turcica sclerosis is minimal (33).

7. Psychogenic Diabetes Insipidus

It is caused by compulsive intake of large amounts of fluid leading to inhibition of normal vasopressin. Obviously, there are no imaging features of this entity. Exclusion of any intracranial lesion by MRI of brain and sella with and without contrast might aid in its diagnosis (2).

8. Nephrogenic Diabetes Insipidus (NDI)

a. **Primary**: It is X-linked recessive condition with unresponsiveness of the tubules and collecting system to vasopressin. For obvious reasons there are no specific imaging features of this entity.
b. **Secondary**: Polycystic kidney disease, drug toxicity such as Lithium toxicity, analgesic nephropathy, reflux nephropathy, amyloidosis, acute tubular nephropathy.

Polycystic kidney disease

Polycystic kidney disease (also known as PKD) is the most common life threatening genetic disorder of kidney can be either autosomal recessive (AR) or autosomal dominant (AD). Both ADPKD/ARPKD are characterized by the development of multiple cysts in both the kidneys, which are often fluid filled leading to increase in size of kidneys.
ADPKD is the most common inherited kidney disease and is postulated to have begun during the embryonic life with fewer than 5% of nephrons being affected at the time of birth. Because of fluid accumulations, cysts continue to grow and cause pressure atrophy of renal parenchyma and worsening of renal failure. Increase in serum creatinine is noted during the second and third decade of life with obvious renal failure during 6th-7th decade of life. Clinical features include abdominal discomfort and pain (most common), hematuria, urinary tract infection, high blood pressure, intracranial bleeding, nephrolithiasis, colon diverticulosis, hepatic cysts, pancreatic cysts, splenic cysts, cysts in seminal vesicle, cardiac cysts, arterial aneurysms (cranial vessels and aorta), abdominal wall hernias, aortic and

mitral valve abnormalities, end stage renal disease, kidney failure and occasionally nephrogenic diabetes insipidus (34-35).

Autosomal recessive PKD (ARPKD) is also called infantile PKD since signs of kidney involvement are often identified even before the birth of child. Children often die within the first few days because of respiratory difficulties arising because of lung hypoplasia secondary to oligohydramnios. In addition, with increasing age, liver scarring is also noted in children.

The diagnosis of PKD is established via imaging (figure 8). Expansile fluid filled cysts of various sizes along with distorted renal cortex and medulla in addition to stretching and elongation of kidney tubules and blood vessels are often noted. Ultrasound is recommended for the initial screening because of ease of performance, easy availability, low cost and no risk of radiation. But, the data obtained with ultrasound is often not reproducible and as accurate as compared to which is obtained via CT or MRI. Occasionally other complications also develop such as infection, hemorrhage, cyst rupture and peritonitis that can also be identified on cross sectional CT or MRI. CT is also useful for volume measurement and assessing structural defects in kidney, however, it involves the use of contrast and radiation.

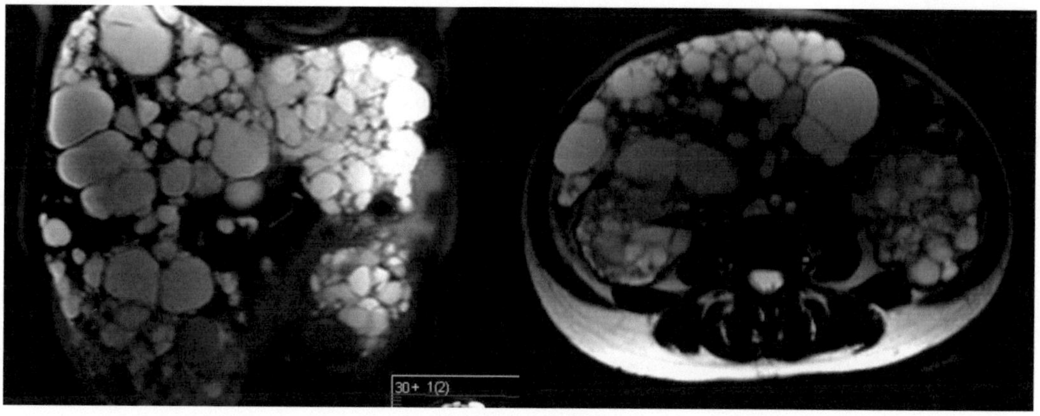

Fig. 8. Coronal HASTE (left) and axial TRUE-FISP (right) MR images show both kidneys completely replaced by cysts appearing as bright rounded structures. Notice non-visualization of any normal renal parenchyma. The patient incidentally also had Polycystic Liver Disease.

Recently, MRI has gained popularity for determining the kidney volume and estimation of disease progression. The data obtained via MRI is often reproducible and accurate in addition to excellent tissue contrast, high resolution 3D images and no need of contrast or radiation. Excellent visualization of renal cyst is obtained via coronal T2 weighted and axial fat saturated T2 weighted imaging showing hyperintense cysts throughout both kidneys. In addition, simple and complex cysts are easily differentiated with T1 weighted imaging. Contrast MRI enable better visualization of renal parenchyma however, use of gadolinium contrast can lead to development of nephrogenic systemic sclerosis in such patients with impaired kidney functions. In addition, MRI also evaluates the blood flow to the affected kidney, which is an important marker of disease progression. With increase in severity of disease, the renal blood flow decreases proportionally. In addition, imaging is also very important based on the reports that combined renal volume is a prognostic indicator of disease severity. CT and MRI are often used for volume measurement over the short period of time whereas in patients with long interval between consecutive follow up, ultrasound is the preferred modality. In addition, other quantitative imaging markers, which are often linked with disease progression, are size, number, spatial distribution, individual growth rate, and asymmetry of cysts. MRI is very often used for measuring and evaluating these markers of disease progression. In addition, family history and genetic testing are also important in diagnosing PKD. In addition, specific anatomic areas can also be evaluated with MRI. Review of literature suggests that kidneys can weigh as much as 8 kg (normal weight is 120-140 gram) secondary to the presence of multiple fluid filled cysts (measuring up o 3 cm) and have length up to 40 cm. In one recent study, it was found that volume of kidney affected by ADPKD was up to 1000 ml (in normal people, mean volume of kidney is 150 ml). Overall, MRI is superior to ultrasonography and CT. MRI efficiently detects small renal cysts as small as 2 mm that are likely to be missed on CT and ultrasound (US). However, MRI is more expensive, less readily available, takes longer time to acquire images and is contraindicated in certain population such as those with pacemakers and other prosthesis. Some of these limitations should be overcome by technical advancements. In addition family history and genetic testing are also used for establishing the diagnosis (34-35).

Lithium nephropathy

Lithium is a well established treatment for affective disorders. It has a narrow therapeutic window, ranging from 0.6 - 1.2 mMol/L. Lithium nephrotoxicity can be classified into nephrogenic diabetes insipidus, acute toxicity, and chronic renal disease. Nephrogenic diabetes insipidus is characterized by polyuria and polydipsia. Mild toxicity can be seen at serum lithium levels of 1.5 - 2.5 mMol/L, with moderate toxicity at levels of 2.5 - 3.5 mMol/L (36).

Lithium toxicity affects multiple organ systems, and may cause coarse tremors, neuromuscular excitability, muscle weakness, sluggishness, nausea, vomiting, diarrhea, and seizures. Rhabdomyolysis can also occur. Decreasing renal function, evidenced by increasing serum creatinine and decreased creatinine clearance, is seen in chronic lithium nephropathy. The only established risk factor is lithium therapy, and an increased duration of therapy increases the risk of progression to end-stage renal disease (ESRD). Discontinuation of lithium therapy does not ensure against progression to ESRD. Chronic lithium nephropathy is a progressive condition, and pathology demonstrates tubular atrophy, glomerulosclerosis, interstitial fibrosis, and distal tubular dilatation with microcyst formation. A recent study found that tubular microcysts were present in 62.5% of renal biopsies performed in patients treated with lithium, involved both the renal cortex and medulla, and measured 1-2 mm in diameter. A serum creatinine level of 2.5 mg/dL at the time of biopsy was found to be the only significant predictor of progression to ESRD (36).

Renal cystic disease is commonly evaluated with US, computed tomography (CT), and MRI. US demonstrates well-circumscribed, anechoic cystic structures with posterior acoustic enhancement, and CT shows hypodense cystic structures measuring between -10 and +20 Houndsfield units (HU). The number and nature of cystic lesions is best characterized by MRI, and T2-weighted imaging most accurately assesses the fluid content of lesions. MRI is a useful tool to evaluate the renal parenchyma, and when combined with magnetic resonance angiography (MRA), can effectively study the renal arteries. T2-weighted images demonstrate the microcysts of chronic lithium nephropathy as small hyperintense 1-2 mm round lesions. In a patient with a history of lithium therapy, MR imaging of abundant microcysts within the kidneys bilaterally strongly supports the diagnosis of chronic lithium nephropathy, and may obviate the need for renal biopsy (36).

Analgesic nephropathy

Analgesic nephropathy is defined as damage to one or both kidneys resulting from chronic exposure to over the counter pain medications such as acetaminophen and NSAIDs or other medications containing phenacetin. It has been suggested that approximately 6 or more pills for 3 years significantly increases the risk for analgesic nephropathy. It is seen in 4 per 100,000 thousand patients and is more common in female above 30 years of age, most of whom are self medicating for relief from chronic pain. It is more common in Europe, Australia and USA. However, its incidence has declined significant in the past few decades owing to decreased consumption of phenacetin containing compounds and public awareness (43-44).

Initial changes include scarring of small blood vessels called capillary sclerosis which in turn lead to renal papillary necrosis and subsequently chronic interstitial nephritis. In the absence of treatment and avoidance of analgesics, patient develops pyelonephritis, renal failure, anemia, high blood pressure, NDI and end stage renal disease. These changes are postulated to result from decrease blood flow to the kidney because of vessel sclerosis and also because of inhibition of prostaglandin E2 production by NSAIDs, depletion of antioxidants and oxidative damage to the kidney.

Both CT and US can be used for assessing kidney damage because of analgesic nephropathy and show bilateral decrease in renal volume combined with either bumpy contours or papillary calcifications. However, US has higher sensitivity than CT scan for detecting RPN due to analgesic nephropathy (37-38).

Reflux nephropathy

Reflux nephropathy (RN) caused because of reflux of urine back into kidneys instead of going forward into the bladder and then into urethra. It is caused because of defective valve at the site of insertion of ureter into bladder and the condition is vesico-ureteric reflux (VUR). Over the period of time, reflux of urine back into kidneys injures the parenchyma and causes small and scarred kidneys. Scarring is almost always seen and often develops within the first five years of life. In addition, patient also develops hypertension, hematuria, proteinuria, chronic renal failure, ESRD and NDI. Recurrent urinary tract infection in male and female children raises the suspicion for RN and warrant further investigations. Initial investigations of choice are ultrasonogram, voiding cystourethrography and renal scientigraphy or nuclear cystography using Tc 99m dimercaptosuccinic acid (DMSA). DMSA scan is now regarded as the most sensitive and specific modality for detecting inflammatory changes within the kidney and also for identifying VUR, particulary the transient episodes and uses low radiation dose. In recent study it was found that DMSA scan was positive in children with negative vesicocysto urethrogram (VCUG), indicating higher sensitivity with DMSA scan. Chronic reflux nephropathy in adult can also be evaluated with IV excretory urography or nephropyelotomography or CT urography, which often reveals calyceal distortion with typical claviform morphology. In addition, dilatation of intra-renal urinary tract is also seen. On voiding cystourethrogram, backward flow of contrast from opacified bladder into the ureter is seen in patients with VUR. In addition, contrast enhanced CT or MRI can also show parenchymal changes such as decrease in renal size and presence of notch of the renal parenchyma surface, parencymal scarring, ureteral dilatation and calyceal clubbing. Long standing reduction in renal mass often leads to glomerular injury and sclerosis. Contrast-enhanced voiding sonocystography is a newer modality and useful alternative. This modality is radiation free and uses microbubble-based contrast agents. Recently, it has been proposed that contrast-enhanced voiding sonocystographyshould be used for both diagnosis and follow up of patients with VUR since several recent studies have shown superiority of Contrast-enhanced voiding sonocystography over VCUG and nuclear cystography for detecting VUR. In addition, MR urography (MRU) is an excellent modality and provides detailed information regarding the anatomy (such as renal contour and caliceal configuration) and functioning of urinary tract. It is suggested that in many ways MRU is more useful than DMSA scan. Recently, Lonergan et al. demonstrated that gadolinium-enhanced inversion-recovery MR imaging has higher sensitivity for detecting focus of infections within the urinary tract and offer greater reproducibility. In addition, MRU provides greater resolution, excellent tissue contrast, detailed analysis of tubular function without causing background artifact and radiation exposure. However, it is an expensive and time consuming modality and requires sedation, which negates its usefulness to some extent (39-41).

Amyloidosis

Amyloidosis is a group of heritable or acquired diseases characterized by the deposition of abnormal proteinacious material as beta-fibrillar sheets in the extracellular space. It can affect almost every organ system either alone or in combination. Primary amyloidosis develop secondary to immune disorder such as multiple myeloma where as secondary amyloidosis is often due to chronic inflammatory diseases such as rheumatoid arthritis. Definitive diagnosis is established with biopsy followed by tissue staining with special dyes. The commonly used staining agent is Congo Red Dye which causes apple green bifringence under polarized light and thioflavine-T (intense yellow-green fluorescence). In addition, imaging can also be crucial for managing patients affected with amyloidosis. Its utility however has been limited due to the fact that imaging findings are often nonspecific and diverse (42-43).

Renal involvement in multiple myeloma (MM) and rheumatoid arthritis (RA) leads to small and contracted kidneys. CT may show either focal cortical mass with focal calcifications or diffuse infiltration in the kidney glomeruli or interstitium. Variability in kidney size reflect the stage of disease. For example, during the acute stage, kidneys may be enlarged with smooth contour whereas in chronic phase kidneys are often shrunken with diffuse irregular contour, thinned cortex and hard texture (called as amyloid contracted kidneys). In addition, diffuse cortical thinning is also noted in chronic phase in addition to focal parenchymal nodules. Other findings noted in renal amyloidosis are amorphous calcification of renal parenchyma, filling defect in renal pelvis either because of blood clot or because of amyloid mass and perinephric mass with calcification. In addition, decreased renal perfusion and reduced elimination of contrast can also be seen on urography and/or angiography in these patients.

On ultrasound, renal amyloidosis often meets the criteria for type 1 renal parenchymal disease. Increase in echogenecity of renal cortex is noted along with medullary prominence which is suggested to be due to the deposition of amyloid, calcium or acute parenchymal diseases. In addition, corticomedullary demarcation is often prominent and arcuate vessels are obscured (42-43).

Recently, it has been suggested that diffusion weighted MRI is also of use in evaluating renal amyloidosis in patient with familial Mediterranean fever. In addition, nuclear scan performed after administration of gallium show enhanced uptake in affected kidneys and is suggestive of disease activity. However, PET/CT failed to show enhanced uptake in case of cardiac and renal amyloidosis (42-44).

Acute tubular necrosis

Acute tubular necrosis or (ATN) is characterized by the death of tubular cells in kidney. Tubular cells constitute kidney tubules, which are key structures for transferring urine to the ureter. These cells also perform reabsorbtion of 99% of water filtered into Bowman's capsule and concentrate the urine. Tubular cells possess regenerating capacity and continuously replace the old and dying cells. This is very important and allows for complete recovery from ATN if precipitating cause is eliminated. ATN often presents with ARF and is the most common cause of ARF. There are two varieties of ATN. One is ischemic ATN and another one in toxic ATN. Ischemic ATN occurs due to decreased perfusion (renal artery stenosis, shock, renal artery emboli) whereas toxic ATN occurs due to exposure to toxins (such as analgesics or antibiotics, hemoglobin, myoglobin, Bence Jones proteins of multiple myeloma, heavy metals, organic solvents, posion and several others). Since the damage occurs to the kidney, it is classified as renal cause of acute renal failure. Urinalysis often shows pathognomonic muddy brown epithelial cast in patients with ATN along with increased fractional excretion of sodium (>3%). Histopathology shows tubulorrhexis, which is a localized necrosis of the epithelial cells lining the renal tubules. In addition, focal rupture or loss of basement membrane is also seen developing skip lesions through the tubules. Due to loss of basement membrane, regeneration is often unlikely in ischemic ATN. In toxic ATN, basement membrane is often intact and allows complete recovery if precipitating cause is removed in timely manner. However, in both types, dead or partially viable cells shed into tubular lumen and lead to obstruction and eventual renal failure. Ultrasound and renal scintigraphy are useful for evaluation and diagnosis of ATN. US show swollen and enlarged pyramids with decreased cortico-medullary differentiation and increased resistive index. On the other hand renal scintigraphy shows normal perfusion, increased retention and decreased excretion (45-46).

9. References

[1] Maghnie M. Diabetes insipidus. Horm Res. 2003;59 Suppl 1:42-54. Review.

[2] Dundas B, Harris M, Narasimhan M. Psychogenic polydipsia review: etiology, differential, and treatment. Curr Psychiatry Rep. 2007 Jun;9(3):236-41.

[3] Maghnie M, Cosi G, Genovese E, Manca-Bitti ML, Cohen A, Zecca S, Tinelli C, Gallucci M, Bernasconi S, Boscherini B, Severi F, Aricò M. Central diabetes insipidus in children and young adults. N Engl J Med. 2000 Oct 5;343(14):998-1007.

[4] Morello JP, Bichet DG. Nephrogenic diabetes insipidus. Annu Rev Physiol.2001;63:607-30.

[5] Bichet DG. Nephrogenic diabetes insipidus. Adv Chronic Kidney Dis. 2006 Apr;13(2):96-104.

[6] Mazumdar A. Imaging of the pituitary and sella turcica. Expert Rev Anticancer Ther. 2006 Sep;6 Suppl 9:S15-22.

[7] Elster AD. Imaging of the sella: anatomy and pathology. Semin Ultrasound CT MR. 1993 Jun;14(3):182-94.
[8] Zee CS, Go JL, Kim PE, Mitchell D, Ahmadi J. Imaging of the pituitary and parasellar region. Neurosurg Clin N Am. 2003 Jan;14(1):55-80, vi.
[9] Arima H, Oiso Y. Mechanisms underlying progressive polyuria in familial neurohypophysial diabetes insipidus. J Neuroendocrinol. 2010 Jul;22(7):754-7.
[10] Carman KB, Yarar C, Yakut A, Adapinar B. Septo-optic dysplasia plus: a patient with diabetes insipidus. Pediatr Neurol. 2010 Jul;43(1):76-8.
[11] McCabe MJ, Alatzoglou KS, Dattani MT. Septo-optic dysplasia and other midline defects: the role of transcription factors: HESX1 and beyond. Best Pract Res Clin Endocrinol Metab. 2011 Feb;25(1):115-24.
[12] Guillemin R. Neuroendocrinology: a short historical review. Ann N Y Acad Sci. 2011 Mar;1220:1-5. doi: 10.1111/j.1749-6632.2010.05936.x.
[13] Sharma RR. Hamartoma of the hypothalamus and tuber cinereum: a brief review of the literature. J Postgrad Med. 1987 Jan;33(1):1-13. Review.
[14] Boyko OB, Curnes JT, Oakes WJ, Burger PC. Hamartomas of the tuber cinereum: CT, MR, and pathologic findings. AJNR Am J Neuroradiol. 1991 Mar-Apr;12(2):309-14.
[15] Levitt MA, Fleischer AS, Meislin HW. Acute post-traumatic diabetes insipidus: treatment with continuous intravenous vasopressin. J Trauma. 1984 Jun;24(6):532-5.
[16] HAY DR. Diabetes insipidus after tuberculous meningitis. Br Med J. 1960 Mar 5;1(5174):707.
[17] Tabuena RP, Nagai S, Handa T, Shigematsu M, Hamada K, Ito I, Izumi T, Mishima M, Sharma OP. Diabetes insipidus from neurosarcoidosis: long-term follow-up for more than eight years. Intern Med. 2004 Oct;43(10):960-6.
[18] Bihan H, Christozova V, Dumas JL, Jomaa R, Valeyre D, Tazi A, Reach G, Krivitzky A, Cohen R. Sarcoidosis: clinical, hormonal, and magnetic resonance imaging (MRI) manifestations of hypothalamic-pituitary disease in 9 patients and review of the literature. Medicine (Baltimore). 2007 Sep;86(5):259-68.
[19] Cunnington JR, Jois R, Zammit I, Scott D, Isaacs J. Diabetes insipidus as a complication of Wegener's granulomatosis and its treatment with biologic agents. Int J Rheumatol. 2009;2009:346136.
[20] Xue J, Wang H, Wu H, Jin Q. Wegener's granulomatosis complicated by central diabetes insipidus and peripheral neutrophy with normal pituitary in a patient. Rheumatol Int. 2009 Aug;29(10):1213-7.
[21] Rivera JA. Lymphocytic hypophysitis: disease spectrum and approach to diagnosis and therapy. Pituitary. 2006;9(1):35-45. Review.
[22] Cemeroglu AP, Blaivas M, Muraszko KM, Robertson PL, Vázquez DM. Lymphocytic hypophysitis presenting with diabetes insipidus in a 14-year-old girl: case report and review of the literature. Eur J Pediatr. 1997 Sep;156(9):684-8.
[23] Dziurzynski K, Delashaw JB, Gultekin SH, Yedinak CG, Fleseriu M. Diabetes insipidus, panhypopituitarism, and severe mental status deterioration in a patient with chordoid glioma: case report and literature review. Endocr Pract. 2009 Apr;15(3):240-5.
[24] Alshail E, Rutka JT, Becker LE, Hoffman HJ. Optic chiasmatic-hypothalamic glioma. Brain Pathol. 1997 Apr;7(2):799-806.

References

[1] IPCC, 2021: Climate Change 2021: The Physical Science Basis. Contribution of Working Group I to the Sixth Assessment Report of the Intergovernmental Panel on Climate Change [Masson-Delmotte, V., P. Zhai, A. Pirani, S.L. Connors, C. Péan, S. Berger, N. Caud, Y. Chen, L. Goldfarb, M.I. Gomis, M. Huang, K. Leitzell, E. Lonnoy, J.B.R. Matthews, T.K. Maycock, T. Waterfield, O. Yelekçi, R. Yu, and B. Zhou (eds.)]. Cambridge University Press. In Pres

[2] World Meteorological Organization (UMO) and UN Office for Disaster Risk Reduction (UNDRR). Climate and Weather-Related Disasters Surge Five Fold Over 50 Years, But Early Warnings Save Lives - WMO Report. UN News, Global perspective Human stories; 2021

[3] World Meteorological Organization. Atlas of Mortality and Economic Losses from Weather, Climate and Water Extremes (1970-2012): WMO,2014

[4] Warm Heart Organization. Climate Change Primer, What Causes Global Warming? Warm Heart Organization; 2021. [Online]. Available from: https://warmheartworldwide.org/climate-change/

[5] Environmental Protection Agency (EPA). Understanding Global Warming Potentials. United States Environmental Protection Agency; 2021. [Online]. Available from: https://www.epa.gov/ghgemissions/understanding-global-warming-potentials [Accessed: 26 November 2021]

[6] The World Green Building Council (WorldGBC), Advancing Net Zero, Ramboll, C40 Cities, "Bringing Embodied Carbon Upfront; Coordinated Action for the Building and Construction Sector to Tackle Embodied Carbon," 2019. (This is an online report available at: https://www.worldgbc.org/sites/default/files/WorldGBC_Bringing_Embodied_Carbon_Upfront.pdf.

[7] GEA, Global Energy Assessment - Toward a Sustainable Future, Cambridge University Press, Cambridge, UK and New York, NY, USA and the International Institute for Applied Systems Analysis, Laxenburg, Austria; 2012

[8] The World Green Building Council (WorldGBC). Global Status Report 2017. UN Environment and the International Energy Agency; 2017

[9] Harvey LDD. Recent advances in sustainable buildings: Review of the energy and cost performance of the state-of-the-art best practices from around the world. Annual Review of Environment and Resources. 2013;**38**:281-309

[10] Holcim Foundation. High Praise for 'Never Demolish' Approach to Sustainable Design. Holcim Foundation; sustainable construction; 2021

[11] Council of Australian Governments (COAG), "Baseline Energy Consumption and Greenhouse Gas Emissions," Department of Climate Change and Energy Efficiency, Australia. 2012

[12] The Guardian Organization, "The Guardian View on Buildings: Out With the New! For the Planet's Sake," The Guardian Opinion Architecture, 2021. [Online]. Available: https://www.theguardian.com [Accessed: 27 November 2021]

[13] Evans D, Liaukus C. Home Renovations Should Be a Climate Change Opportunity. Bloomberg; 2021. [Online].

Available: https://www.bloomberg.com/news/articles/2021-11-10/home-renovations-should-be-a-climate-change-opportunity. [Accessed: 27 November 2021]

[14] Torcellini P, Pless S, Deru M, Crawley D. Zero energy buildings: A Critical Look at the Definition. Golden, CO (United States): National Renewable Energy Lab. (NREL); 2006

[15] Carpino C, Loukou E, Heiselberg P, Arcuri N. Energy performance gap of a nearly Zero Energy Building (nZEB) in Denmark: The influence of occupancy modelling. Building Research and Information. 2020;**48**(8):899-921

[16] Pless S, Torcellini PEP. Getting to net zero. ASHRAE Journal. 2009;**51**(9):18

[17] The European Parliament and the Council of the European Union, "EPBD, Directive 2002/91/EC of the European Parliament and of the Council of the 16th of December 2002 on the Energy Performance of Buildings", Official Journal of the European Communities, 2002. Available at: https://eur-lex.europa.eu/LexUriServ/LexUriServ.do?uri=OJ:L:2003:001:0065:0071:EN:PDF

[18] The European Parliament and the Council of the European Union, "EPBD recast, Directive 2010/31/EU of the European Parliament and of the Council of the 19th of May 2010 on the Energy Performance of Buildings (Recast)." Official Journal of the European Communities; 2010. Available at: https://eur-lex.europa.eu/LexUriServ/LexUriServ.do?uri=OJ:L:2010:153:0013:0035:EN:PDF

[19] Lindholm O, Reda F. Positioning positive energy districts in European cities. Buildings. 2021;**11**(1):19

[20] Biggs J. Six Low-Carbon Building Materials for a Greener Construction Industry. Procore; 2021. [Online]. Available from: https://www.procore.com/ [Accessed: 26 November 2021]

[21] Architecture 2030. Carbon Smart Materials Palette – Actions for Reducing Embodied Carbon at Your Fingertip. 2030 Palette. Architecture 2030 Project. Santa Fe, New Mexico, United States. [Online]. Available: https://materialspalette.org [Accessed: 26 November 2021]

[22] Cheshire D, Burton M. The Carbon and Business Case for Choosing Refurbishment Over New Build. AECOM; 2021. [Online]. Available: aecom.com [Accessed: 26 November 2021]

[23] Energy Vanguard, "Air Leakage Results at Elevated Pressure - Energy Vanguard," Energy Vanguard Blog; 2021. [Online]. Available: https://www.energyvanguard.com [Accessed: 26 November 2021]

[24] Zero Energy Project. Super-Insulate the Net Zero Building Envelope. [Online]. Available: https://zeroenergyproject.org/build/twelve-steps-affordable-zero-energy-home-construction-design/super-insulate-net-zero-building-envelope [Accessed: 22 November 2021]

[25] National Fenestration Rating Council. What Higher Energy Performance Means for Your Home; Windows, Doors, and Skylights. NFRC; 2020. [Online]. Available: https://www.nfrc.org/windows-doors-skylights/ [Accessed: 26 November 2021]